Crohn's Disease
Your Questions • Expert Answers

Andrew S. Warner, MD
Chairman, Department of Gastroenterology
Lahey Clinic
Burlington, MA

Amy E. Barto, MD
Director, Inflammatory Bowel Disease Center
Lahey Clinic
Burlington, MA

JONES & BARTLETT
L E A R N I N G

Burlington, Massachusetts

BOSTON　　TORONTO　　LONDON　　SINGAPORE

World Headquarters
Jones & Bartlett Learning
5 Wall Street
Burlington, MA 01803
978-443-5000
info@jblearning.com
www.jblearning.com

Jones & Bartlett Learning books and products are available through most bookstores and online booksellers. To contact Jones & Bartlett Learning directly, call 800-832-0034, fax 978-443-8000, or visit our website, www.jblearning.com.

The authors, editor, and publisher have made every effort to provide accurate information. However, they are not responsible for errors, omissions, or for any outcomes related to the use of the contents of this book and take no responsibility for the use of the products and procedures described. Treatments and side effects described in this book may not be applicable to all people; likewise, some people may require a dose or experience a side effect that is not described herein. Drugs and medical devices are discussed that may have limited availability controlled by the Food and Drug Administration (FDA) for use only in a research study or clinical trial. Research, clinical practice, and government regulations often change the accepted standard in this field. When consideration is being given to use of any drug in the clinical setting, the healthcare provider or reader is responsible for determining FDA status of the drug, reading the package insert, and reviewing prescribing information for the most up-to-date recommendations on dose, precautions, and contraindications, and determining the appropriate usage for the product. This is especially important in the case of drugs that are new or seldom used.

Production Credits
Executive Publisher: Christopher Davis
Managing Editor, Special Projects: Kathy Richardson
Production Assistant: Leia Poritz
Manufacturing and Inventory Control Supervisor: Amy Bacus
Composition: Northeast Compositors, Inc.
Cover Design: Carolyn Downer
Cover Image: Top left photo: © Jason Stitt/ShutterStock, Inc.; Top right photo: © Edyta Powlowska/ShutterStock, Inc.; Bottom photo: © Alexander Raths/ShutterStock, Inc.
Printing and Binding: Malloy, Inc.
Cover Printing: Malloy, Inc.

ISBN: 978-1-4496-5623-2

6048

Printed in the United States of America
15 14 13 12   10 9 8 7 6 5 4 3 2

Contents

Crohn's disease is one of the most common forms of inflammatory bowel disease (IBD). Believed to be caused by an autoimmune process, Crohn's disease is characterized by chronic inflammation of the gastrointestinal tract, and potentially of many different organ systems throughout the body. Symptoms of inflammatory bowel disease range from mild to severe, and up to three-quarters of patients with Crohn's disease eventually need surgery. Fortunately, many effective treatments are currently available, with new and potentially even more effective therapies on the horizon.

This book is intended to be a patient-oriented, practical guide about Crohn's disease. The questions have been taken from thousands we have been asked over the years by patients with IBD. The answers are a compilation of the latest scientific information along with our own experience in treating inflammatory bowel disease. In essence, this book recreates a visit to the healthcare provider's office. It contains the questions you wished you had asked and many that you never thought to ask. We explore how inflammatory bowel disease is diagnosed and treated, complications of the disease including dysplasia and cancer, when to have surgery and the different types of operations performed, diet and nutrition, lifestyle, and reproductive issues and pregnancy. This book can provide you with important and useful information, as well as an in-depth understanding of the many facets and nuances of Crohn's disease.

PART ONE

The Basics

What are Crohn's disease and inflammatory bowel disease?

How do you get Crohn's disease?

Is Crohn's disease contagious?

More . . .

1. What are Crohn's disease and inflammatory bowel disease?

Crohn's disease is one of the most common forms of inflammatory bowel disease (IBD). Although the cause of IBD is unknown, it appears to be a result of disruption in the normal functioning of the **immune system**. In Crohn's disease the immune system attacks the gastrointestinal system, which is the digestive tract or tube in the body that runs from the mouth to the **anus** (see **Figure 1**). Crohn's disease may simultaneously involve different areas of the **gastrointestinal tract**, with dis-

Crohn's disease

An intestinal disease characterized by chronic intestinal inflammation; can affect any area of the gastrointestinal tract.

Immune system

An internal network of organs, cells, and structures that work to guard your body against foreign substances, such as infections.

Anus

The outside opening of the rectum.

Gastrointestinal tract

The digestive tube that starts at the mouth and ends at the anus.

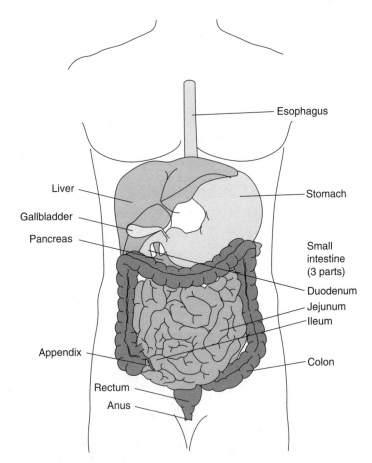

FIGURE 1 Normal gastrointestinal anatomy.

eased segments of intestine alternating with normal segments. As a result, the intestines become chronically inflamed—red, raw, and swollen—a condition often accompanied by intestinal ulcers, **fistulas**, and **abscesses**. This ongoing **inflammation** can lead to a variety of symptoms, including abdominal discomfort, diarrhea, rectal bleeding, fever, and weight loss. In Crohn's disease a certain **cell** called a **granuloma** appears on occasion (which is why Crohn's disease is also called **granulomatous enteritis** or **granulomatous colitis**).

Crohn's disease covers a wide spectrum of severity. Some Crohn's disease patients become very ill and debilitated, whereas others have symptoms that are mild and easier to control. Crohn's disease can also affect the joints, skin, and eyes and can lead to **malabsorption** and weight loss, **kidney stones**, **gallstones**, and many other ailments. The vast majority of individuals with Crohn's disease need to take medication regularly, and up to 70% to 80% of Crohn's disease patients eventually undergo surgery.

2. How do you get Crohn's disease?

Crohn's disease is considered to be a type of **autoimmune** disease. Normally, the immune system functions like a defense system, guarding our bodies against attack from foreign agents—bacteria, **cancer**, viruses, and parasites, to name a few. An autoimmune disease occurs when the body's immune system becomes confused and starts attacking normal organs and cells, believing that they are foreign. We don't know why this happens. One theory proposes that IBD is triggered by an infection, such as a bacteria or virus, with the inflammation continuing even though the infection has long

THE BASICS

Fistula

A tunnel connecting two structures that are not normally connected; examples include a fistula between the rectum and vagina (rectovaginal fistula) or the colon and bladder (colovesicular fistula).

Abscess

A walled-off collection of pus; in Crohn's disease, an abscess is most commonly found around the anus or rectum, but can occur anywhere in the body.

Inflammation

A process characterized by swelling, warmth, redness, and/or tenderness; can occur in any organ.

Cell

The smallest unit in the body; millions of cells attached together make up the organs and tissues.

Granuloma

A certain type of cell found in Crohn's disease; can also be seen in other, nongastrointestinal diseases.

Granulomatous enteritis

Crohn's disease of the small bowel.

Granulomatous colitis

Crohn's disease of the colon.

Malabsorption

A condition in which the small intestine is not able to absorb nutrients and vitamins.

Kidney stones

Stones that form in the kidneys.

Gallstones

Stones that form in the gallbladder.

Autoimmune

An inflammatory process in which your immune system attacks part of your own body, such as the colon in ulcerative colitis.

Cancer

An uncontrolled growth of cells in the body that can form a tumor and can spread, or metastasize, to other areas of the body.

Immune dysregulation

Failure of the body to appropriately regulate the immune system; this lack of regulation is believed to be integral to the development of Crohn's disease and ulcerative colitis.

Genetic predisposition

An inherited trait that makes one more likely to develop a disease.

since healed. This is known as **immune dysregulation**, or a failure of the body to regulate the immune system appropriately. Many of the drugs used to control Crohn's disease focus on modulating or suppressing the immune system. Also, some people have a **genetic predisposition** to develop Crohn's disease; research in this area is in its earliest stages.

If you have Crohn's disease, it is important for you to realize that you did nothing to cause yourself to develop it and you could have done nothing to prevent it. It's not from something you ate or didn't eat; it's not from drinking too much alcohol or coffee; it's not from stress, working too hard, or lack of sleep. We simply do not know what causes Crohn's disease. What we do know is how to diagnose and treat it.

3. Is Crohn's disease contagious?

No. Crohn's disease is not contagious.

4. What is IBD and why is it called that?

Inflammatory bowel disease, or IBD, is an intestinal disease characterized by chronic inflammation; Crohn's disease and ulcerative colitis are the two most common forms.

5. Is IBD the same thing as IBS?

No. Although there is only a one-letter difference in their names, IBD (inflammatory bowel disease) and **IBS (irritable bowel syndrome)** are two entirely distinct and different disorders. IBD is considered an intestinal disease. IBS, on the other hand, is what is known as a functional disorder (see **Table 1**). A functional disorder is not a true disease but rather a collection of subjective symptoms, such as diarrhea and abdominal pain, with no actual objective abnormalities found. So, while the subjective symptoms of IBD and IBS are similar, the distinction is that with IBD, objective abnormalities are found by laboratory, radiologic, or endoscopic testing, whereas with IBS the results of all tests return normal. This is not to say that IBS is not an actual disorder or that it's just in someone's head. IBS, much like a migraine headache, does have actual, physical symptoms, but without any objective findings it cannot be classified as a disease. So, then, what is it?

IBS, as mentioned, is a functional disorder characterized by abdominal discomfort, diarrhea or constipation, sometimes diarrhea alternating with constipation, or a combination of these symptoms. Individuals with IBS are often classified as being pain-predominant, diarrhea-predominant, or constipation-predominant, depending

Irritable bowel syndrome (IBS)

A functional disorder characterized by atypical abdominal pain, diarrhea, constipation, diarrhea alternating with constipation, the feeling of incomplete fecal evacuation, or any combination of these symptoms.

THE BASICS

TABLE 1 Characteristics of IBS

Functional disorder
No objective abnormalities
Subjective symptoms
Atypical abdominal pain
Irregular bowel habits • Diarrhea • Constipation • Diarrhea alternating with constipation
Urgent bowel movements
Feeling of incomplete evacuation

upon the predominant symptom. The abdominal pain can be across the entire abdomen, or localized to one area of the abdomen (often the lower right or lower left side). However, some individuals with IBS may have just right upper side abdominal pain with no other symptoms. And although diarrhea is a common symptom, if one were to measure the total quantity of stool produced by someone with IBS over a 24-hour period, he or she would find that the actual stool volume was well within normal limits. So while subjectively a person with IBS may experience loose stool, the stool volume is actually normal. (Diarrhea is medically defined by stool volume and not stool consistency.) Along the same lines, individuals with constipation usually have normal **colonic transit time**, which is the amount of time it takes stool to travel from the beginning of the colon to the rectum. (Colonic transit time is determined by a test called a stool marker study. In this relatively easy-to-perform test, the patient ingests a capsule filled with approximately 20 radio-opaque markers that can be seen on a simple abdominal X-ray. If after 5 days most of the markers are still in the colon, the patient has a delay in colonic transit. If no markers are present, the patient's colonic transit is normal. Colonic transit time is usually normal in people with IBS.)

Like IBD, IBS is a chronic disorder, and individuals with IBS learn to make appropriate lifestyle modifications. Because stress often exacerbates IBS, stress reduction is an integral part of therapy. Avoiding aggravating foods, such as fried and fatty foods, and caffeinated beverages is equally critical. If lifestyle modification alone does not control symptoms, individuals with IBS can take various drugs such as intestinal antispasmodics. However, unlike IBD, the mainstay of therapy for

Colonic transit time

The time it takes for stool to travel from the beginning of the colon (the cecum) to the rectum.

IBS should be lifestyle and dietary modification and not pharmacologic therapy. Patients with IBS don't usually develop IBD, but patients with IBD often experience IBS-type symptoms. IBD patients who suffer from IBS-type symptoms often experience relief with treatment aimed at the IBS symptoms.

6. How do you know if you have Crohn's disease?

Crohn's disease can be varied in the way it presents itself. As a result, Crohn's disease may be difficult to diagnose because it can be easily confused with other disorders. Crohn's disease can involve any area of the gastrointestinal tract and symptoms are mostly determined by which area of the digestive tract is affected.

The ileum is involved in approximately 70% of patients with Crohn's disease—40% the ileum alone and 30% the ileum and cecum combined. Patients whose Crohn's disease affects this location usually present symptoms of pain in the right lower side of the abdomen, especially after eating, and often have abdominal **distention** (bloating). Diarrhea and weight loss may also be seen. At times, the ileum can become narrowed to the point that the patient can develop a bowel **obstruction**.

Crohn's disease is limited to the colon (no ileum, or small bowel involvement) in about 20% of patients. Also called Crohn's colitis, abdominal cramps and non-bloody diarrhea are usually the presenting symptoms. While ulcers in the colon are found in Crohn's disease, little or no rectal bleeding occurs in Crohn's colitis.

Distention

Abdominal bloating usually from excess amounts of gas in the intestines; can be a sign of a bowel obstruction.

Obstruction

A blockage of the small intestine or colon.

CROHN'S DISEASE: YOUR QUESTIONS • EXPERT ANSWERS

In individuals whose Crohn's disease is diffusely spread throughout the small bowel, cramps, diarrhea, and weight loss usually are the major symptoms. If the disease is severe, malabsorption accompanied by significant weight loss can also be seen. Individuals whose Crohn's disease involves the stomach and duodenum experience upper abdominal pain, nausea, and vomiting as the predominant symptoms, much as they would experience if they had an ulcer.

Sometimes it can be difficult to distinguish between Crohn's disease and other disorders, such as ulcerative colitis. This situation may occur when Crohn's disease involves the rectum and colon and presents with symptoms much like those of ulcerative colitis. In such a case, potential ways to distinguish between the two diseases include the following:

- Small bowel involvement—may be seen in Crohn's disease and is never seen in ulcerative colitis.
- Appearance of ulcers on **colonoscopy**—Crohn's disease ulcers tend to be discrete and are often very deep, whereas ulcerative colitis ulcers are more confluent and superficial.
- **Biopsy**—Crohn's disease has granulomas; ulcerative colitis does not.
- Fistulas and **perianal** abscesses—can be seen in Crohn's disease and are almost never found in ulcerative colitis.
- Blood testing—Crohn's disease is more likely to test positive for anti-Saccharomyces cerevisiae antibody (ASCA), whereas ulcerative colitis is more likely to test positive for antineutrophil cytoplasmic antibody (ANCA).

Colonoscopy

An endoscopic procedure in which a small, thin, flexible lighted tube with a camera on the end is passed through the rectum into the colon and, at times, into the ileum; an excellent test to detect inflammation and strictures in the rectum, colon, and ileum, and one that allows for a biopsy to be taken.

Biopsy

Usually performed during an endoscopy, a small piece of mucosa (inside lining of the intestine) is removed and examined under a microscope; an excellent test to characterize types of inflammation and detect dysplasia and cancer.

Perianal

The area adjacent to the outside of the anus; common site for abscess and fistula formation.

7. Can someone have Crohn's disease and not know it?

It is not at all uncommon for someone to have Crohn's disease without knowing it. In fact, most Crohn's patients have symptoms for months to years before they seek help. In these cases, the symptoms are usually mild enough so as not to interfere with the individual's ability to go about a daily routine.

8. How common is Crohn's disease?

Crohn's disease is not a common disease. Currently, it is estimated that approximately 1.6 million people in the United States have some form of IBD. The incidence of Crohn's disease has risen over time, although it is unclear whether this is due to a true increase in number of people with Crohn's disease or simply better recognition of the disease. Currently, the **prevalence** (the number of people affected by a disease in a population at a specific time) of IBD is around 75 to 150 cases per 100,000 people. Crohn's disease is more commonly found in developed countries and in northern latitudes, and is less commonly found in less industrialized countries and in more temperate climates. Also, Crohn's disease is more often seen in urban settings and is less frequently found in more rural environments.

Prevalence

The number of people affected by a disease in a population at a specific time.

The peak onset of Crohn's disease usually occurs in late adolescence and extends to early adulthood (ages 15 to 30 years), but a person can be diagnosed with the disease at any age—from 5 to 85 years. Crohn's disease seems to occur equally in males and females and occurs more often in those of Jewish decent, with Ashkenazi Jews having the highest prevalence.

THE BASICS

9. What role does inflammation play in Crohn's disease?

Chronic inflammation—meaning long-term soreness, irritation, and swelling of the gastrointestinal tract—is the main characteristic of Crohn's disease. In fact, in 1932, Drs. Burrill Crohn, Leon Oppenheimer, and Gordon Ginzburg first described Crohn's disease as inflammation of the terminal ileum (lower end of the small intestine) and called the disease "regional enteritis" or "terminal ileitis." We now know that Crohn's disease can occur anywhere in the gastrointestinal tract, particularly the small intestine, the colon, or both. Without the presence of this intestinal inflammation, your gastroenterologist may suspect you have a condition other than Crohn's disease, such as irritable bowel syndrome (IBS).

When your body has Crohn's disease, molecules released by the immune cells in response to a perceived threat to the immune system cause inflammation in the lining of the gastrointestinal tract, which can lead to ulceration, and ultimately scarring (also called fibrosis). The inflammation can be felt as abdominal discomfort or diarrhea, which can range from mild in some individuals to severe in others.

10. Is inflammation responsible for my symptoms?

The inflammation of Crohn's disease is responsible for the abdominal discomfort you feel and can also cause other symptoms. Unlike some other immune inflammatory diseases, inflammation in Crohn's disease can affect all layers of the gastrointestinal tract. This chronic inflammation can lead to the development of sores, called ulcers, along the intestinal lining. Because the ulcers from Crohn's disease can penetrate the entire wall of the intestine, a fistula and/or abscess can develop. Fistulas are abnormal tunnels or connections between two adjacent organs. Fistulas can occur between organs, such as the bladder and bowel (called enterovesical), rectum and vagina (rectovaginal), or one loop of bowel and a neighboring loop of bowel (enteroenteric). External fistulas can develop between the intestine and the skin (enterocutaneous). Fistulas develop in between 20% and 40% of patients with Crohn's disease.

Chronic inflammation can also cause scar tissue to build up in the gastrointestinal tract over time and may cause a stricture to develop.

It is important, however, to note that inflammation does not affect just the lining of the gastrointestinal tract. The inflammatory cells circulating in the body can cause many other symptoms that may seem unrelated to the gastrointestinal inflammation. Question 35 addresses these other symptoms.

11. If I can reduce the inflammation, will I get better?

While Crohn's disease is a lifelong disorder, the good news is that there are medications available to help treat the inflammation of Crohn's. Treating the inflammation along with learning how to modify your diet and lifestyle has allowed many individuals with Crohn's disease to enjoy a full and productive life. This may mean monitoring your symptoms, changing your diet, reducing stress in your life, or talking to your gastroenterologist about maximizing treatment to reduce inflammation.

12. Am I more likely to get colon cancer if I have Crohn's disease?

Individuals with Crohn's disease that primarily affects the colon are considered to be at higher risk for colon cancer than the general population. However, because in Crohn's disease less of the colon is usually involved than in other disorders such as ulcerative colitis, the overall likelihood that a Crohn's disease patient will develop colon cancer is less than that of an ulcerative colitis patient.

Primary sclerosing cholangitis

Inflammation and scarring of the bile ducts within the liver; can occur in ulcerative colitis and Crohn's disease.

Additional risk factors are **primary sclerosing cholangitis**, which is a liver disorder that is associated with Crohn's disease, family history of colon cancer (immediate relation), and, possibly, activity of disease. It should also be clearly stated that although individuals with Crohn's disease that primarily affects the colon are considered to be at increased risk, this is as compared to the general population in which the chance of getting colon cancer in a person's lifetime is approximately 1 in 20. Although having Crohn's disease (if it primarily affects the colon) does place you at increased risk as compared to someone who does not have Crohn's disease, the majority of Crohn's disease patients still will not develop colon cancer.

Individuals with Crohn's disease may experience an increased incidence of lymphoma and small bowel cancer. However, because these are rarely found, it is difficult to determine how frequently lymphoma and small bowel cancer actually occur.

13. Can I do anything to prevent getting colon cancer?

Some scientific evidence indicates that long-term medical therapy with aminosalicylates may reduce the likelihood of developing colon cancer in patients with inflammatory bowel disease (although more specifically, ulcerative colitis). It is thought that chronic suppression of inflammation may inhibit the transformation of normal cells into **dysplastic cells**. Although the available data regards only aminosalicylates, many healthcare providers extend these findings to immune-modulating therapy as well. Also, there are some suggestions in the medical literature that nutritional therapy with folic acid and calcium may be protective, but this is "softer" data and the results may simply be based on chance occurrence. However, it may be advisable to take a daily multivitamin containing folic acid and calcium.

THE BASICS

Dysplastic cells

Cells that are in a state of abnormal growth or development.

PART TWO

Diagnosis

How is Crohn's disease diagnosed?

Is Crohn's disease ever confused
with other disorders?

Can I ever be cured of Crohn's disease,
or will I have it for my entire life?

More . . .

14. How is Crohn's disease diagnosed?

No one test can definitively diagnose someone as having Crohn's disease with 100% certainty. Crohn's disease is diagnosed based upon a patient's clinical history and physical examination in combination with radiologic, endoscopic, and laboratory testing. And because each patient is an individual, not all patients undergo an identical evaluation; testing is tailored to each patient. Following is a description of some of the various tests that are used in the evaluation of Crohn's disease.

Radiology

- **Abdominal X-ray**: Provides a picture of structures and organs in the abdomen and is helpful in detecting a bowel obstruction or **perforation**.

Perforation

A rupture or abnormal opening of the intestine that allows intestinal contents to escape into the abdominal cavity.

Duodenum

The first part of the small intestine just beyond the stomach.

- **CT scan**: Uses **X-rays** to create a more detailed look inside the body. A computed tomography (CT) scan is especially helpful in detecting an abscess and also is useful in evaluating for inflammation, bowel obstruction, or perforation.
- **Upper GI series/upper GI series with small bowel follow-through**: Allows a close examination of the esophagus, stomach, **duodenum**, and small bowel. The patient must drink a thick, white liquid barium shake, and then is x-rayed as the material travels through the gastrointestinal tract. This is an excellent test to help detect strictures, fistulas, and inflammation in the stomach and small bowel.
- **Enteroclysis**: Provides a detailed examination of the small bowel by passing a small tube through the nose, into the stomach, and into the duodenum; barium is then introduced through the tube directly

into the small bowel. This is an excellent test to help detect minor abnormalities in the small intestine that might not be seen on an upper GI series with small bowel follow-through.

- **Barium enema**: Allows a close examination of the rectum and colon by introducing barium through the rectum and taking X-rays as it travels through the colon. This is an excellent test to help detect strictures, inflammation, and fistulas in the colon.
- **Ultrasound**: Uses sound waves to examine abdominal and pelvic organs; commonly used to look for gallstones and obstruction of the bile duct.
- **MRI**: Uses a magnetic field to create a detailed picture of the structures and organs in the abdomen and pelvis. Magnetic resonance imaging (MRI) is especially helpful in detecting abdominal and pelvic abscesses; it can also be used to evaluate the **bile duct** and pancreatic duct.
- **Virtual colonoscopy**: A CT scan of the colon. This radiologic examination technique is still in the early stages of development but shows promise as a method to detect colon abnormalities.

Endoscopy

Endoscopy is a broad term that includes a variety of endoscopic tests, including **upper endoscopy** and colonoscopy. Prior to an endoscopic procedure, the patient receives a set of instructions describing the procedure in detail, including any preparations that may need to be made. All endoscopic procedures require a period of fasting beforehand. Some procedures require a colon prep, which involves flushing out the colon by way of liquid laxatives and ingestion of lots of fluids.

Bile duct

A channel through which bile flows from the liver to the intestines.

Upper endoscopy

A procedure in which a small, thin, flexible, lighted tube with a camera on the end is passed through the mouth into the esophagus, stomach, and duodenum; an excellent test to detect inflammation and strictures in the upper gastrointestinal tract that allows a biopsy to be taken.

17

Most, but not all of these procedures are performed under **sedation**, which is administered intravenously. The sedatives do not make a patient completely unconscious, but rather induce a twilight state in which the patient is comfortable and sleepy. A patient will often entirely forget that the procedure has taken place and will wake up at the end of the procedure asking, "When are you going to get started?"

Each of the following procedures (except capsule endoscopy) is performed using an endoscope (in the case of colonoscopy, the tool is called a colonoscope; see **Figure 2**). An endoscope is a small, thin, flexible tube (about the width of a finger) with a light and a camera mounted on the end of the tube that is inserted through the mouth or, in the case of a colonoscope, the rectum. The physician can take a biopsy by using a set of forceps passed through a thin channel in the endoscope. The forceps removes a tiny piece of tissue that is then sent to a lab for examination under a microscope by a **pathologist**. This type of biopsy is routine and is painless.

Potential complications of endoscopic procedures include perforation of the bowel and bleeding. These risks

Sedation

Also called conscious sedation, or moderate sedation; sedation is a form of moderate anesthesia in which the patient is given medication to induce a state of relaxation. Patients under sedation are sleepy and are less likely to feel discomfort.

Pathologist

A physician trained in the evaluation of organs, tissues, and cells, usually under a microscope; assists in determining and characterizing the presence of disease.

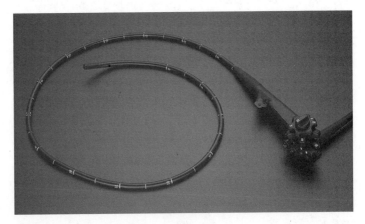

FIGURE 2 A colonoscope.

are very small, and the complications are correctable. Although these procedures can be anxiety provoking, many are routine and are performed by most **gastroenterologists** on a daily basis.

Following are descriptions of the individual endoscopic procedures:

- **Upper endoscopy:** The endoscope is passed through the mouth into the esophagus, stomach, and duodenum. This is an excellent test to help detect inflammation and strictures in the upper gastrointestinal (GI) tract and allows for a biopsy to be taken.
- **Colonoscopy:** The colonoscope is passed through the rectum into the colon and, sometimes, into the ileum. This is an excellent test to detect inflammation and strictures in the rectum, colon, and ileum and allows for a biopsy to be taken.
- **Sigmoidoscopy:** This procedure is performed with or without sedation; this is a "short" version of the colonoscopy and is used to examine the rectum and the first third (left side) of the colon.
- **Proctoscopy:** This procedure is performed without sedation, usually on a special tilt table that positions the patient with his or her head down and buttocks up. In this procedure, a rigid, straight, lighted tube is used to examine the rectum. Although this procedure has mostly been replaced by flexible sigmoidoscopy, it is still an excellent test to examine the rectum.
- **Anoscopy:** This procedure is performed without sedation, usually on a special tilt table that positions the patient with his or her head down and buttocks up. In this procedure, a rigid, short, straight, lighted tube is used to examine the anal canal. This is an excellent test to examine for an anal fissure or hemorrhoids.

Gastroenterologist

A physician who specializes in diseases of the gastrointestinal tract, liver, and pancreas.

DIAGNOSIS

- **Enteroscopy:** This procedure is performed while the patient is under sedation. A small, thin, long, flexible, lighted tube with a camera on the end, the enteroscope, is passed through the mouth into the esophagus, stomach, duodenum, and jejunum. This is an excellent test to detect inflammation and strictures in the upper GI tract and upper small intestine. The type of endoscope used for an enteroscopy is called an enteroscope and is longer than a traditional endoscope; thus, it can look deeper into the small intestine.

- **Capsule endoscopy:** This procedure is performed without sedation. The patient swallows a large pill containing a camera and wears a sensor device on the abdomen. The capsule passes naturally through the small intestine while transmitting video images to the sensor, which stores data that can be downloaded to a computer for your gastroenterologist to review. Because the capsule can travel where traditional endoscopes can't reach, this test is mostly used in evaluating patients with chronic gastrointestinal bleeding of obscure origin. While capsule endoscopy can also be used to evaluate for Crohn's disease of the small bowel, other simpler tests are usually adequate and often more accurate in diagnosing and assessing the extent and severity of the disease. In addition, the capsule, which is very large, can easily become lodged in an intestinal stricture and cause an obstruction for which the patient would then need an operation to remove the capsule.

- **ERCP:** This endoscopic procedure is performed under sedation and is used to examine the bile duct and pancreatic duct. This procedure is performed for a variety of reasons, including detecting and removing stones in the bile duct, to detect tumors involving the bile duct and pancreatic duct, and to diagnose primary sclerosing cholangitis. ERCP (endoscopic retrograde cholangiopancreatography) can also be used to dilate and place stents across strictures in the bile duct and pancreatic duct.

Histology

- **Biopsy**: Usually performed during an endoscopy. A small piece of mucosa (the inside lining of the intestine) is removed and examined under a microscope. This is an outstanding test to characterize types of inflammation and detect dysplasia and cancer.

Laboratory Testing

Through the use of blood tests, your gastroenterologist can determine whether you are anemic, malnourished, vitamin deficient, have electrolyte imbalances, or have other abnormalities that could contribute to your symptoms. Some evidence indicates that testing positive for anti-Saccharomyces cerevisiae antibody (ASCA) suggests that a patient has Crohn's disease. This laboratory test is not routine and is not usually necessary to establish a diagnosis of Crohn's disease.

Stool Testing

Stool tests are performed to rule out an infection as the cause for intestinal symptoms. Even individuals with long-standing Crohn's disease may need occasional stool testing because an infection can arise and its symptoms can mimic those of Crohn's. Stool testing can also be helpful in determining causes of malabsorption.

Breath Testing

Breath testing can be performed to look for **lactose intolerance** and **bacterial overgrowth** as possible causes for your symptoms.

Lactose intolerance

The inability to absorb dairy products caused by a deficiency of the lactase enzyme; a type of malabsorption disorder.

Bacterial overgrowth

A condition in which an overgrowth of normal intestinal flora occurs; usually seen in the setting of an intestinal stricture.

15. Is Crohn's disease ever confused with other disorders?

Because the symptoms of Crohn's disease are often nonspecific and can occur in many different diseases, they are frequently confused with other gastrointestinal disorders. For example, diarrhea, which is one of the most common symptoms of Crohn's disease, can occur in many other intestinal disorders—infectious **gastroenteritis**, such as traveler's diarrhea or giardiasis; dietary causes, such as lactose intolerance or drinking too much coffee or tea; **celiac sprue**, a malabsorption disorder; an overactive thyroid; and laxative abuse. Chronic or recurrent abdominal pain may also be caused by a myriad of dysfunctions, such as gallbladder disease, **pancreatitis**, or a stomach ulcer. Rectal bleeding can occur with hemorrhoids, an anal fissure, and colon cancer. Weight loss may occur as a result of many of the conditions listed here and may also be seen with other diseases, including pancreatic cancer, **anorexia**, and **bulimia**. Last, individuals with irritable bowel syndrome often have a combination of diarrhea and abdominal pain.

Because the symptoms of Crohn's disease are nonspecific, a gastroenterologist may perform various radiologic and endoscopic tests to help make the correct diagnosis. However, sometimes even the tests do not give clear-cut answers. For example, infectious gastroenteritis may look almost identical to Crohn's disease because colonic ulcers can occur in both disorders. And because ulcers also occur in both **peptic ulcer disease** and Crohn's disease of the stomach and duodenum, these conditions can often be confused as well. Since many other diseases may mimic Crohn's disease, gastroenterologists often order several tests to help establish a firm diagnosis.

Gastroenteritis

An intestinal illness characterized by abdominal cramps and diarrhea; usually caused by an infection.

Celiac sprue

A malabsorption disorder characterized by intolerance to gluten, which is a protein found in wheat, barley, rye, and sometimes nuts.

Pancreatitis

Inflammation of the pancreas; most often caused by gallstones, alcohol use, or as a drug side effect.

Anorexia

An eating disorder in which someone does not want to eat and has an unrealistic fear of gaining weight.

Bulimia

An eating disorder in which someone induces vomiting after eating, sometimes after eating large amounts of food, which is termed binging and purging.

Peptic ulcer disease

The condition in which an ulcer forms in the stomach or duodenum; may be from acid or the bacteria *Helicobacter pylori*.

Diverticulosis is another disease that can be confused with colonic Crohn's disease, colon cancer, or **colonic ischemia** (a condition in which the colon becomes damaged from a lack of blood flow). Diverticulosis consists of tiny **benign** sac-like protrusions or outpouchings in the colon. (Each single sac is called a diverticulum; together as a group they are called diverticulosis.) These protrusions occur in the muscular wall of the colon, often at sites that are slightly weakened by the natural penetration of small arteries. Diverticulosis is thought to be due to tension on the wall of the colon as produced by gas and stool. This condition is more often seen in Westernized, industrialized countries like the United States, and is likely a consequence of our relatively low-fiber American diets. Diverticulosis can happen anywhere in the colon, but in most situations it starts in the left side of the colon and may progress throughout the colon over time. These tiny pockets are most readily seen in the lining of the colon during a colonoscopy, barium enema, or CT scan. Once diverticulosis develops, it never goes away. One way to help prevent diverticulosis is to eat a high-fiber diet. This helps to bulk up the stool and keeps it moving through the colon. High fiber foods might include wheat or multigrain breads, fiber cereals, fresh fruits, and vegetables.

Diverticulosis becomes more common as we get older, affecting approximately 5% of people at age 40 years, 30% at age 60 years, and up to 65% of people age 85 years. Sometimes younger people can have diverticulosis, though this is less common. Diverticulosis most commonly starts in the left side of the colon, but in young people it can occur more predominantly in the right side of the colon. The vast majority of people with diverticulosis are never bothered by it and may not know they have it unless it is discovered during a

Colonic ischemia

Colon inflammation caused by lack of blood flow; also called ischemic colitis.

Benign

A noncancerous growth.

DIAGNOSIS

colonoscopy. Two potential problems can happen in the setting of diverticulosis—these tiny pockets can bleed, and they can become infected (called diverticulitis, as discussed next). Approximately 5% to 15% of people with diverticulosis may develop bleeding, and 15% to 25% of patients may develop diverticulitis.

Diverticular bleeding, as mentioned, is uncommon. Bleeding occurs as the diverticulum expands and stretches, causing injury to the small artery, which runs alongside it. Due to the very thin wall of the diverticulum pocket and the closeness of the artery, the artery can sometimes rupture into the diverticulum and cause bleeding. Symptoms usually consist of maroon stools or bright red blood per rectum. These symptoms often happen abruptly, with people feeling like they suddenly need to use the bathroom. They rush to the toilet, and proceed to expel a large volume of bright red blood that gushes into the bowl. Sometimes people think they've had a loose stool, but looking at the toilet bowl, they see only blood, or a good amount of blood mixed with a small amount of maroon stool. Rarely do people experience abdominal pain, except for some slight cramping when they are just about to move their bowels. The bloody bowel movements can occur several times in quick succession, often prompting people to rush to the emergency room.

Understandably, this type of abrupt-onset rectal bleeding can be very frightening. However, the majority of people stop bleeding on their own, and rarely is the bleeding life-threatening. Those who take additional blood thinners may have more pronounced bleeding than others. People are often admitted to the hospital for observation and blood transfusions. They may undergo a colonoscopy to document the existence of underlying diverticulosis as the cause of the bleeding, but usually the bleeding has already stopped and it is quite uncommon to find an actively bleeding diverticulum. Because there are usually multiple diverticulum pockets in the colon, the gastroenterologist usually cannot tell which one was the culprit for the bleeding. Furthermore, if someone comes to the hospital with abrupt-onset, painless, bright red blood per rectum, and a history of a previous colonoscopy showing diverticulosis, the gastroenterologist may not need to repeat a colonoscopy, but rather will observe the person in the hospital until the bleeding has stopped.

In rare cases, the bleeding persists and additional tests performed by a radiologist can help to localize and potentially stop the bleeding. These tests are called a **tagged red blood cell scan** and an angiogram. Both require active bleeding to be helpful in finding the source of the bleeding. A tagged red blood scan involves the injection into an IV of radiologically "tagged" red blood cells. These are then watched on a nuclear scan to see into which area of the colon these tagged red blood cells leak and collect in pools. An angiogram, which requires a slightly faster pace of bleeding, involves injecting dye directly into the large arteries of the colon (through a needlestick into an artery in the neck or groin, similar to a cardiac catheterization) and watching where the dye leaks out and pools at the site of bleeding. An angiogram is additionally helpful because medications can be injected right at the site of bleeding to scar down the artery, or a plug can be inserted into the bleeding artery to do the same.

In the majority of patients, diverticular bleeding stops on its own. For those cases where the bleeding does not

Tagged red blood cell scan

A radiologic procedure done on patients who are actively bleeding internally, but the exact location of the bleeding is unclear.

stop, or stops and starts multiple times within the same hospitalization, surgery to remove the affected portion of the colon may be necessary. If the diverticulosis is limited to the left side of the colon, then often removal of the left colon and reattachment of the two healthy ends of colon (without needing a colostomy bag) can be performed. For those who have diverticulosis through-out the colon and the site of bleeding cannot be clearly localized, the entire colon may need to be removed.

Up to 20% of people can have recurrent diverticular bleeding. This can happen at any time, from the day they leave the hospital up to years later. While this in-formation may not seem reassuring to those who have had a diverticular bleeding episode, it is important to remember that most people do not bleed again. Because no one can predict if and when the bleeding might hap-pen again, it is important to go on with life as normal. If the bleeding does happen again, the symptoms will be similar to the first bleeding episode, and one should have a plan of action ready to return immediately to the nearest hospital for further evaluation and treatment.

Diverticulitis involves inflammation and subsequent infection of an individual diverticulum. Lots of people mistakenly use the terms diverticulosis and diverticuli-tis interchangeably, but in reality these similar sound-ing terms mean very different things. It is the "ITIS" portion of the word diverticulitis that means infection/inflammation, just like other terms such as appendicitis or meningitis. Diverticulitis occurs when a food particle or small piece of stool gets stuck in a diverticulum, caus-ing erosion, and damage to the inner lining. This leads to inflammation with a tiny "micro" perforation (or hole) in the colon wall, which quickly becomes infected with local bacteria, leading to a small collection of pus, or abscess, in that area of the colon. Symptoms of diverticulitis include fever and abdominal pain, most often in the left lower part of the abdomen. Other symptoms include nausea, vomiting, diarrhea, and constipation. Rectal bleeding in association with diverticulitis is rare. A healthcare provider will usually find tenderness upon examining the belly, and there will often be an elevated white blood cell count by laboratory testing. A CT scan of the abdomen is not usually necessary to make the diagnosis, but can confirm the diagnosis by visualizing the infected area of colon along with adjacent abscess.

Depending on how sick a person is, he or she may be admitted to the hospital for bowel rest, intravenous hydration, and intravenous antibiotics. Others may be sent home on a combination of two oral antibiotics. Most people get better quickly, although severe cases of diverticulitis may require immediate surgery, and rarely can result in complications, including stricturing (narrowing) of the colon, communications (fistulas) involving other organs in the pelvis such as the bladder, and obstruction (or blockage) of the colon. During the recovery phase, you should stick to a low-fiber diet to allow the colon to rest and heal without increasing the amount of undigested roughage moving through it.

After a bout of diverticulitis, some gastroenterologists may caution patients to avoid all nuts and corn/popcorn, as well as foods containing seeds such as strawberries and tomatoes. The theory is that these food particles are what become lodged in a diverticulum and cause trouble. There is a good deal of controversy among healthcare providers about this topic. We recommend ingesting these foods in moderation. If someone can link his/her episode of diverticulitis to eating a large amount of one of these foods, then he/she would do best to avoid eating this food excessively in the future. Going crazy trying to cut out all seeds and nuts in the diet is likely not worth the effort, nor is it scientifically proven.

One thing that a person can do to try and prevent further episodes of diverticulitis is to increase the amount of fiber in his/her diet. As mentioned above, this should be done only after the episode of diverticulitis is fully healed. Fiber can come from many sources, including fresh fruits and vegetables, fiber-rich cereals, and multigrain and wheat bread. It is important to know that increasing fiber in the diet can lead to either a temporary or persistent increase in symptoms such as bloating, abdominal cramping, and excess gas. Big gas producers include broccoli, cauliflower, cabbage, Brussels sprouts, and beans. Adding fiber, especially for those not used to it, should be done slowly to allow the body to adjust. Fiber supplements can also be helpful to regulate bowel movements and promote overall colon health. Fiber supplements with a higher degree of synthetic versus organic fiber may cause less of the symptoms noted above.

Anyone who has a bout of diverticulitis should undergo a colonoscopy to ensure that nothing else caused the inflammation in the colon, including less likely diagnoses such as Crohn's disease or colon cancer. The colonoscopy is often performed at least six to eight weeks later to allow for proper healing of the colon. Once the underlying diverticulosis is identified and no other abnormalities are found, then the gastroenterologist can be assured that diverticulitis was the likely diagnosis.

Surgery is sometimes offered to remove the portion of the colon containing diverticulosis to prevent further episodes of diverticulitis. This option is often discussed with people who have had recurrent bouts of diverticulitis, or those who have had a severe episode. For some people, this issue might be brought up after a first bout of diverticulitis. Surgery is usually offered because once diverticulitis happens repeated episodes can be more severe. Once diverticulitis happens twice, the chance of it happening again gets higher with each episode. The question of whether to undergo surgery, as well as how many repeat episodes should pass before surgery is performed, needs to be decided on an individual basis.

16. Can I ever be cured of Crohn's disease, or will I have it for my entire life?

Unfortunately, Crohn's disease is chronic and usually a lifelong disease; therefore, it is a disease from which you can never be completely cured. Fortunately, however, both improved diagnostic capabilities and advances in treatment enable the vast majority of individuals with Crohn's disease to be treated successfully. Patients can enjoy long periods of **remission** in which they are symptom free. From time to time, you may meet someone who states that he or she once had Crohn's disease but is now "cured" and has been free of symptoms and off medication for years—such patients are few and far between. Crohn's disease is a chronic disease and individuals should expect to remain on some form of long-term therapy to maintain control of their symptoms.

Remission

The state of having no active disease. It can refer to clinical remission, meaning no symptoms are present; endoscopic remission, meaning no disease is detected endoscopically; or histologic remission, meaning no active inflammation is detected on biopsy.

17. Can I die from having Crohn's disease?

Although Crohn's disease is a chronic disease, it is exceedingly unlikely that you will die from having it. The vast majority of patients with Crohn's disease are able to enjoy long and rewarding lives filled with work, family, friends, and leisure, no different from anyone else. Much like someone who has learned to live with the aches and pains of **arthritis**, individuals with Crohn's disease are able to enjoy life by learning how to work around the limitations of their disease.

Arthritis

Inflammation of the joints; individuals with arthritis often have pain, redness, tenderness, and swelling in the affected joints.

PART THREE

Complications

I have a friend with Crohn's disease who was operated on for a bowel obstruction. Does this occur often in Crohn's disease?

What is a stricture?

I heard that people with Crohn's disease can get something called a fistula. Can you tell me what this is?

More . . .

18. I have a friend with Crohn's disease who was operated on for a bowel obstruction. Does this occur often in Crohn's disease?

Crohn's disease is characterized by chronic intestinal inflammation, which can cause scar tissue to form within the intestinal tract. Over time, this process of inflammation leading to scarring may cause a segment of the intestinal tract to become narrowed; this is called a stricture or **stenosis**. The stricture can become progressively narrowed to the point of completely obstructing the intestinal tract. Another way the intestine can become blocked is when acute inflammation develops on top of a stricture, causing the intestine to become swollen. When the intestinal track becomes obstructed, it is also called a bowel obstruction (**Table 2**). An additional way for a bowel obstruction to develop is if a patient with an intestinal stricture eats something that is difficult to fully digest, such as raw vegetables. This could potentially plug up the stricture and lead to an obstruction. Nuts, berries, popcorn, and unripe fruit are also known to do this.

Strictures in the small bowel are best seen with an upper GI small bowel series or with an enteroclysis, which is an advanced type of small bowel series. Strictures in the

Stenosis

A stricture, or narrowing; in Crohn's disease, often a narrowing of the bowel.

TABLE 2 Major Complications Associated with Crohn's Disease

Obstruction
Perforation
Hemorrhage
Sepsis
Fistula
Abscess
Toxic megacolon

colon can be diagnosed with either a barium enema or colonoscopy; virtual colonoscopy, which is a CT scan of the colon, may also show a stricture. A bowel obstruction is usually easily visualized on a simple abdominal X-ray; a CT scan of the abdomen can also be used and often provides additional information, such as the cause of the obstruction.

When a bowel obstruction occurs, patients usually experience intense abdominal pain, abdominal distention, little or no passage of stool or gas, and sometimes vomiting. Individuals in this scenario are almost always hospitalized both for treatment of the obstruction, as well as for monitoring for complications, such as an intestinal perforation. Treatment consists mostly of not eating or drinking anything so as not to worsen the obstruction, intravenous fluids for hydration, and intestinal decompression with nasogastric suction (a small, **nasogastric tube** is passed through the nose into the stomach and then is connected to a suctioning device). Intravenous corticosteroids are sometimes given as well. The majority of patients respond to this therapy.

Those who do not respond to therapy usually require surgery to relieve the obstruction. This type of surgery frequently involves resecting the segment of bowel that is obstructed. In another type of operation, rather than resecting the stricture, the surgeon opens up or widens the stricture, which is called a **strictureplasty**. This latter type of operation, however, is usually not performed in the setting of an emergency operation in a patient with a bowel obstruction. Strictureplasty is mostly done as an elective operation in a patient who may have multiple strictures and for whom the surgeon wants to limit the amount of bowel removed.

Nasogastric tube

A long, flexible tube that is passed through the nose into the stomach and is used to suction out the stomach in the setting of a bowel obstruction or sometimes after an operation.

Strictureplasty

An operation to open up an intestinal stricture.

A bowel obstruction can also develop as a result of an **adhesion**. An adhesion is the presence of scar tissue that has formed inside the **abdominal cavity** but outside of the intestines themselves. Adhesions are mostly seen after a prior abdominal operation of any type, such as appendectomy or hysterectomy, and are not particular to just Crohn's disease. The treatment of a bowel obstruction from an adhesion is similar to that of an intestinal stricture: eating and drinking nothing, intravenous hydration, and nasogastric suction. Intravenous corticosteroids would be of little benefit in this setting.

When a patient with active Crohn's disease who also has had a prior abdominal operation presents with a bowel obstruction, it is often difficult to tell whether it is from an intestinal stricture or an adhesion. Fortunately, the treatment is similar for both problems and the majority of patients heal without the need for surgery.

19. What is a stricture?

An intestinal stricture, or narrowing, is a partial blockage of the bowel that is commonly found in Crohn's disease. A stricture can develop from active intestinal inflammation, leftover scarring from prior inflammation, or a combination of the two. Small bowel strictures are best diagnosed with an upper GI small bowel series (an X-ray with swallowed barium), whereas colonic strictures are more easily seen with a colonoscopy or barium enema (an X-ray with barium injected into the rectum).

Adhesion

Scar tissue that forms internally, usually after an operation; a common cause of bowel obstruction.

Abdominal cavity

The part of the body below the chest and above the pelvic bone that contains the internal organs, including the small intestine, colon, stomach, liver, pancreas, kidneys, and bladder.

20. I heard that people with Crohn's disease can get something called a fistula. Can you tell me what this is?

A fistula is a small tunnel or channel that forms between two structures in the body that are normally not connected. In Crohn's disease, the most common type of fistula is a perianal fistula. A perianal fistula is when a tunnel forms between the lower rectum and the skin surrounding the anus. In women, fistulas may also form between the rectum and vagina. This is called a rectovaginal fistula. Other types of fistulas include fistulas between two sections of the small bowel (enteroenteric fistula), between the small bowel and the colon (enterocolonic fistula), between two parts of the colon (colocolonic fistula), between the colon and the bladder (colovesicular fistula), and between the small bowel and skin (enterocutaneous fistula). The reason a fistula may form is because in Crohn's disease the inflammatory process often involves the full thickness of the bowel wall. The inflamed bowel may then adhere to a nearby structure, such as the rectum to the vagina. In such a case, a small tunnel or fistula may develop between the two adherent structures.

The type of fistula and degree of symptoms determine what treatment is most appropriate. Fistulas between intestinal segments are mostly asymptomatic and are usually not treated beyond standard therapy for Crohn's disease. Perianal fistulas, rectovaginal fistulas, and colovesicular fistulas, on the other hand, usually cause a wide range of symptoms. Small, mildly symptomatic fistulas are usually treated with antibiotics. Complex and debilitating fistulas may require more intensive drug therapy with biologic therapy. Also, surgical techniques are often employed in treating complex fistula disease. On rare occasion, a **colostomy** or ileostomy may be required to divert the fecal stream away from the fistulas to give the fistulas a better chance of healing.

21. What is an anal fissure?

An anal fissure is a small cut or tear that can be seen in the anal canal. Although small, an anal fissure can be very painful because the anus is extremely sensitive. Typically, you might experience a burning pain during or after a bowel movement and often find a streak of blood coating the stool and on the toilet paper. Anal fissures are seen most often when someone with constipation strains to have a bowel movement and passes a hard stool, which creates a superficial tear in the anal canal. Anal fissures can also occur with diarrhea; the constant bowel activity and frequent wiping traumatizes the area. For acute treatment of an anal fissure, you can apply a cortisone/anesthetic cream or a topical nitroglycerine ointment; if severe, Botox injections may also be used. In the long term, better regulation of your underlying bowel pattern to avoid both constipation and diarrhea is the best treatment.

Anal fissures are commonly seen in patients with Crohn's disease. In the setting of Crohn's disease, an anal fissure may represent active Crohn's disease in the anus itself. As such, anal fissures complicating Crohn's disease are usually more resistant to treatment than an anal fissure in someone who does not have Crohn's disease. The initial treatment for an anal fissure in an individual with Crohn's disease is similar to the treatment in someone without Crohn's disease, as described earlier. If the anal fissure does not respond, additional drug therapy with antibiotics, immune-modulating or biologic agents may be employed. Less commonly, anal surgery may be indicated.

22. I have Crohn's disease and often get abscesses around my rectum. What exactly is an abscess and how is it treated? Can I get abscesses in other places?

An abscess is a localized infection, or collection of pus, that your body has walled off, much like a pimple. An abscess can form at any site in the body, but in Crohn's disease it is most often seen around the rectum and anus and is referred to by various names—anorectal abscess, perianal abscess, or perirectal abscess. In an anorectal abscess, the infection arises in the tissue surrounding the anus and rectum. Patients often experience a throbbing and constant rectal pain that is exacerbated when sitting. They may also feel a lump around the anus. If the abscess spontaneously drains, a fistula may be formed. The most common sites of drainage are around the anus (perianal fistula), and in a woman, into the vagina (rectovaginal fistula). Fistulas can track under the skin to more distant sites, such as the scrotum in a man and the vulva in a woman. To prevent these more complex fistulas from forming, surgical drainage may need to be performed. While a fistula to the skin might still develop at the site of the surgical drainage, it is likely to be less debilitating than a fistula to the vagina, vulva, or scrotum. Antibiotics are usually prescribed as well.

Colostomy

Surgically created connection between the colon and the skin to allow for the diversion of fecal material; the waste empties into a bag attached to the skin.

COMPLICATIONS

Some individuals can develop a deeper abscess around the rectum. In these patients, the abscess usually has a more insidious presentation with deep rectal or lower abdominal discomfort, back pain, and/or fever and absence of a palpable lump around the anus. This type of abscess can often be identified by a rectal exam. Because a rectal exam in this situation may be extremely painful, not infrequently patients are taken to the operating room to have a rectal exam after being anesthetized, which is called an EUA, or **evaluation under anesthesia**. At the same time, the surgeon can also incise and drain the abscess without causing the patient any discomfort. In addition to draining the abscess, the surgeon may decide to place a wick or drain in the abscess to allow it to slowly heal from the inside out. Otherwise, the abscess might close superficially on the skin side without fully closing internally, thus allowing for the potential that the abscess will re-form. The surgeon may also choose to place a **seton**, a small, thin, flexible piece of plastic tubing that is inserted through the skin and into the abscess, out the abscess, into the rectum, and then out through the anus where the two ends are tied together. This is usually performed in the case of a large or recurring abscess to allow for long-term drainage so as to prevent the abscess from re-forming. The seton can be left in place for weeks to months and can be easily removed in the office after the drainage has stopped.

Other modalities used to diagnose a deep abscess include a CT scan, MRI, and endorectal ultrasound.

Sometimes a chronic abscess or fistula may develop. In these cases, the patient may be given chronic antibiotics, often for many months. In addition, immune-modulating or biologic agents are often prescribed.

Evaluation under anesthesia (EUA)

Physical examination of the rectum and peri-rectal area performed when the patient is anesthetized; usually done to evaluate for an abscess and/or fistula.

Seton

A small, thin, flexible piece of tubing that is inserted through the skin, into an abscess, out of the abscess, into the rectum, and then out through the anus where the two ends are tied together.

PART FOUR

Surgery

What is the role of surgery in Crohn's disease?

What types of operations are performed
in Crohn's disease?

How often does Crohn's disease recur after
surgery, and is there any way to prevent it?

More . . .

23. What is the role of surgery in Crohn's disease?

Although Crohn's disease is usually adequately treated with medical therapy, approximately 70% to 80% of patients will still need to undergo surgery at some point in their lifetime. Surgery becomes necessary when medical treatment is no longer able to keep the symptoms of Crohn's disease under control, or when a complication arises.

When a person's Crohn's disease is no longer responsive to medical therapy, the decision to perform surgery should be made jointly by you, your gastroenterologist, and your surgeon. To achieve the best outcome, all three parties should be in agreement. Often, you may want surgery because you are frustrated by your illness and feel that you won't get better. However, your physicians may encourage you to be patient, knowing from experience and extensive training that the medicine might need more time to work fully. In addition, because Crohn's disease has such a high postoperative **recurrence** rate, gastroenterologists are often reluctant to recommend surgery until all reasonable medical options have been exhausted. At other times, however, a gastroenterologist may recommend surgery knowing that there are no good medical options left, while you may not yet be ready psychologically for an operation. One of the many factors that physicians take into account when deciding on surgery is whether you are on any medication that either has caused or has the potential to cause you harm.

When a complication occurs, the decision to have surgery is more clear-cut. If a bowel perforation, bowel obstruction, toxic megacolon, sepsis, or an abscess de-

Recurrence

The reappearance of a disease.

velops, surgery is almost always indicated. This is not to say that nonoperative therapy might not be attempted, but that the threshold to operate is much lower and the decision is usually made much quicker.

24. What types of operations are performed in Crohn's disease?

In Crohn's disease, the most common type of operation performed is to surgically remove the diseased segment of intestine, which is known as a bowel resection. The two healthy ends of intestine are then sewn or stapled together to form what is called an **anastomosis**, which is a surgical connection between the two structures. Sometimes, an anastomosis cannot be created; if this is the case, an ileostomy or colostomy may be required. An ileostomy is when the surgeon brings the small bowel (usually the ileum) through the abdominal wall and attaches it to the skin. The end of the ileum is made to protrude through the skin to form what is called a **stoma**. A colostomy is when the colon is used in place of the ileum. Waste products are then collected into an external pouch, or bag (see **Figure 3**). One of the main reasons that an ileostomy or colostomy is formed rather than an anastomosis is the presence of an intra-abdominal infection (i.e., infection within the abdominal cavity). If the anastomosis were to become infected, it could break down and leak bowel contents into the abdomen. This could cause peritonitis, an even more severe intra-abdominal infection. Therefore, rather than run this risk, the surgeon may choose to create an ileostomy or colostomy until the initial intra-abdominal infection has resolved. Then, at a later time, the surgeon will perform a second operation to take down the ileostomy or colostomy and form an anastomosis

Anastomosis

A surgically made connection between two structures in the body; in Crohn's disease, this is usually between two segments of intestine after a resection, or between the intestine and the skin to create an ileostomy or colostomy.

Stoma

The surgically created opening where the intestine or colon meets the skin in an ileostomy or colostomy, respectively.

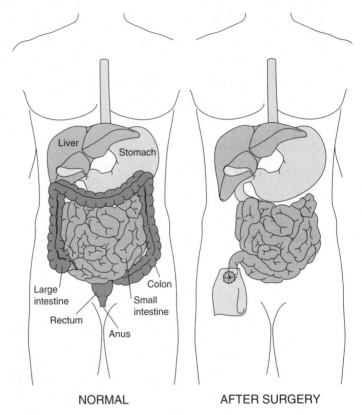

FIGURE 3 Normal anatomy (L); Ileostomy with external bag (R).

between the two remaining sections of bowel. At times, however, it may be necessary to have a permanent ileostomy or colostomy.

A colostomy is sometimes created in the setting of severe perianal Crohn's disease. When a patient becomes debilitated from recurrent perianal abscesses and fistulas that do not heal with maximal medical therapy, a colostomy may be formed to divert the fecal stream away from the rectum and anus. This improves the chances that the abscesses and fistulas will heal because the area is no longer bathed with stool. Unfortunately, once the colostomy is taken down and bowel continuity restored, the abscesses and fistulas often recur. For this reason, a diverting colostomy created to protect the perianal area is often permanent.

Strictureplasty is another operation commonly performed in Crohn's disease. In this operation, the surgeon widens or opens up a small bowel stricture to relieve the patient of obstructive symptoms. Strictureplasty is often referred to as bowel-preserving surgery because the diseased bowel is not removed. This allows patients to preserve more of their intestines. Usually, the surgeon decides to perform a resection versus a strictureplasty during the operation based upon the operative findings.

Intestinal **bypass** is an operation for Crohn's disease that is less commonly performed today. In this operation, rather than resect the diseased segment of intestine, the surgeon bypasses the bowel by connecting the healthy intestine above the diseased segment to the healthy intestine below. As an example, for ileal Crohn's disease, the surgeon would bypass the Crohn's disease by connecting the healthy intestine above the diseased ileum to the healthy colon below. Unfortunately, some patients developed cancer in the bypassed segment of intestine, which is why this operation is now almost never performed.

Bypass

An operation in which a segment of diseased intestine is bypassed by connecting the healthy intestine above the diseased segment to the healthy intestine below.

25. How often does Crohn's disease recur after surgery, and is there any way to prevent it?

One of the most frustrating aspects of Crohn's disease is that it can never be completely cured. After undergoing intestinal resection and creation of an anastomosis, the vast majority of patients have their Crohn's disease recur. Interestingly, when an ileocolic resection (removal of the lower ileum and first part of the colon, the most common operation for Crohn's disease) is performed for Crohn's disease of the ileum, recurrence of Crohn's disease is almost always found above the anastomosis on the small bowel side; it is unusual for Crohn's disease to recur below or on the colon side of the anastomosis. On the other hand, when the ileocolic resection is done in the setting of Crohn's disease involving the colon, the recurrence can be seen on either or both sides of the anastomosis. Also, Crohn's disease tends to follow patterns. If the patient had a short stricture in the ileum before surgery, the recurrence after surgery will probably be a short stricture as well. The reason that Crohn's disease behaves in such a predictable fashion after surgery has never been understood.

What is the rate of postoperative recurrence? After a resection, approximately 20% of patients develop symptoms of Crohn's disease at 2 years, 30% at 3 years, and 50% at 5 years. This is also called the clinical recurrence rate. The endoscopic recurrence rate is much higher. If a colonoscopy was performed on every patient after surgery, signs of a recurrence could be found in up to 70% in 1 year and 85% in 3 years. The frequency of recurrence after an ileostomy is much lower--about 10 to 20% at 10 years. However, once the ileostomy is reversed and an anastomosis is created, the recurrence rate increases.

Is there any way to prevent a recurrence? If we could make only one recommendation, it would be to stop smoking. Cigarette smoking significantly increases the risk of a recurrence; quitting smoking reduces this risk. Any decision to recommend postoperative prophylactic drug therapy in hopes of preventing or delaying a recurrence must be made on an individual basis. In an individual who has had extensive or multiple intestinal resections, prophylactic therapy with an aminosalicy-late or immune-modulating drug may be reasonable. On the other hand, in an individual who has had only a single, limited resection, postsurgical prophylactic therapy may offer only marginal benefit.

SURGERY

PART FIVE

Diet and Nutrition

I find that if I watch what I eat and eliminate certain foods, I feel better. Does that mean that Crohn's disease is caused by something in the diet and can be cured by eating the right types of food?

Is Crohn's disease caused by a food allergy?

How does having Crohn's disease affect my nutrition?

More . . .

26. I find that if I watch what I eat and eliminate certain foods, I feel better. Does that mean that Crohn's disease is caused by something in the diet and can be cured by eating the right types of food?

The causes of Crohn's disease are not known, but research has yet to prove that it is caused by something in the diet. This is not to say that diet does not play a role in this disease—it does. What you eat always has an impact on how you feel. Limiting your diet to foods that do not cause intestinal upset would make anyone feel better. This type of dietary modification is helpful for any type of intestinal problem, not just for Crohn's disease. What is clear is that in Crohn's disease, modifying your diet does not have an effect on the actual underlying inflammation. If you are temporarily unable to eat certain foods while in a flare or recovering from a flare, this is simply a status check that the body is not ready yet.

Though foods can't treat or flare Crohn's disease, choosing the right foods can help you deal better with the symptoms of these diseases, like abdominal pain, bloating, and diarrhea. For example, patients with Crohn's disease who have intestinal strictures are less likely to experience a bowel obstruction if they avoid foods that are hard to digest fully, such as salads, raw fruit and uncooked vegetables, dried fruits, nuts, berries, corn, and even popcorn. Milk products can be problematic for a variety of people with Crohn's disease. Lactose intolerance is caused by a deficiency of the **lactase** enzyme, which is found normally in the small intestine. Individuals with Crohn's disease may be prone to lactose intolerance as a result of inflammation and damage to

Lactase

The intestinal enzyme responsible for the breakdown of lactose; deficiency in this enzyme leads to lactose malabsorption.

the lining of the small intestine, which interfere with lactose absorption. Many patients report improvement in their symptoms simply after they stop eating at fast-food restaurants. So, although Crohn's disease is not caused by anything in the diet, paying attention to what you eat can still help you feel better.

Some people get frustrated and feel like they can't eat anything they consider "healthy." Don't despair—sometimes small changes can be very helpful. For example, if you like fresh fruits/vegetables, you might substitute apples and pears with ripe banana, applesauce, and soft melon. Many vegetables can be cooked thoroughly and pureed. Always beware of big gas producers like broccoli, cauliflower, cabbage, beans, and Brussels sprouts. Often, once your Crohn's disease is under control, you can carefully expand your diet to include some foods you used to enjoy. A nutritionist is a vital member of your medical team and can help you with food choices and menu planning. He or she can also make sure you are not restricting your diet too much and missing out on vital nutrients.

27. Is Crohn's disease caused by a food allergy?

No. No scientific evidence links Crohn's disease to food allergies. The vast majority of adults who believe that they have an allergy to food are actually suffering from **food intolerance**, or intolerance to the method by which the food is prepared. The difference between **food allergy** and food intolerance is that a food allergy is caused by an immune system reaction, whereas intolerance does not involve the immune system. Lactose intolerance is a common example of a food intolerance.

Food intolerance

An adverse reaction to food that does not involve the immune system.

Food allergy

An immune system response to a food that the body mistakenly believes is harmful.

Allergies to tree nuts, peanuts, cow's milk, eggs, soy, fish, and shellfish are the most common true food allergies. Children often outgrow allergies to cow's milk, eggs, and soy. Those who are allergic to tree nuts, peanuts, fish, and shellfish usually remain allergic for life.

What should you do if you believe you are intolerant of a certain food? The most obvious measure is to eliminate that food from your diet and see if you feel better. Common sense dictates that if a food doesn't agree with you, avoid it! As mentioned earlier, certain foods are best avoided during a flare of Crohn's disease. So, although many people often wonder whether gastrointestinal diseases are related to true food allergies, few, if any, are.

28. How does having Crohn's disease affect my nutrition?

Most of the foods that you eat are broken down in the stomach and absorbed in the small intestine. Many disorders can affect the small intestine and interfere with its ability to absorb nutrients properly. When this occurs, it is called malabsorption. The nutrients that may be malabsorbed include a wide variety of food breakdown products such as carbohydrates, fats, and proteins. Other essential dietary elements can also be affected, including iron, calcium, zinc, vitamin B_{12}, folate, and the fat-soluble vitamins A, D, E, and K.

Malabsorption can cause a variety of symptoms. If severe, it can cause weight loss, fatigue, and diarrhea. The diarrhea is often described as foul smelling, with greasy stools that may float in the toilet bowl (called **steatorrhea**), become difficult to flush, and leave an "oil slick"

Steatorrhea

The presence of excess fat in the stool.

on the surface of the water. These changes in stool are often caused by malabsorption of fat, which can be measured in the stool. Again, these types of symptoms are often found only in the later stages of severe malabsorption. Most individuals with malabsorption may have only mild symptoms or no symptoms at all. Sometimes the only sign of malabsorption is the presence of anemia or a vitamin deficiency.

Individuals with Crohn's disease that involves the small bowel often have some level of malabsorption, whether it is obvious by symptoms or shows up only on blood tests. This is because over time inflammation of the small bowel can cause damage to the intestinal lining, which interferes with the absorption of food products. Your gastroenterologist is always on the lookout for signs of malabsorption and may order blood tests routinely to ensure that you do not develop major vitamin or nutrient deficiencies. Patients with Crohn's disease can develop anemia caused by iron, folate, or B_{12} deficiencies. Two other very important nutrients are calcium and vitamin D. Malabsorption of these nutrients, which can potentially lead to osteoporosis, can be found in individuals with small bowel Crohn's disease or anyone with Crohn's disease who takes long-term corticosteroids.

Individuals who have had portions of their small bowel surgically removed may suffer from malabsorption because of the simple fact that there is less small bowel available for absorption of nutrients. If enough small bowel is removed, patients can develop short bowel syndrome (also called **short gut syndrome**). This is mostly seen in patients who have had Crohn's disease for many years and who have had multiple surgeries

Short gut syndrome

A condition of severe malabsorption caused by extensive small bowel resection.

from which less than 100 cm of small bowel remains. These individuals have a very tough time keeping up with absorption of food and fluids, and they can easily become malnourished or dehydrated.

Total parenteral nutrition (TPN)

Nutrition supplied intravenously.

Patients who have short bowel often need additional intravenous nutrition in the form of **total parenteral nutrition**, or **TPN**. TPN is administered on a daily basis through a permanent IV line that is surgically placed into a deep vein to allow for a high concentration of nutrients to be administered; small, superficial veins, such as those on the hands and arms, are too frail to withstand the daily infusion of highly concentrated nutrition. Patients are taught to self-administer TPN at home, usually over 10 to 12 hours at night. Nationwide companies exist solely to provide home nutrition and employ teams of nurses and medical assistants specially trained to provide the necessary support right in your home. If you are on home TPN and want to go on vacation, the "bags" of TPN can be delivered wherever you go. Although this may sound drastic, individuals on long-term home TPN can live happy, healthy, and independent lives.

What is the difference between malabsorption and malnutrition? As stated earlier, malabsorption occurs when the small intestine loses its ability to absorb the nutrients and vitamins from the food that you eat. Malnutrition is an end result of malabsorption, when your body is unable to take in enough nutrients to maintain good health. Malnutrition can also happen if you don't eat enough or eat only junk foods.

29. *How do I know if I should take vitamins?*

Eating a healthy diet is sound advice for anyone wanting to maintain good health. For individuals with Crohn's disease, following this advice can, at times, prove to be challenging. Patients with Crohn's disease often live with dietary restrictions that make it difficult to eat a well-balanced diet. Because vitamins come from the various food groups, eating a restricted diet may reduce the intake of the recommended daily allotment of vitamins. Therefore, anyone who is on a restricted diet should take a daily multivitamin to supplement what he or she may be missing.

Selective vitamin deficiencies can also occur in Crohn's disease. This is more commonly found in people with small bowel Crohn's disease than it is in colonic Crohn's disease because absorption of vitamins occurs mostly in the small bowel. Vitamin B_{12} is absorbed in the ileum. Accordingly, vitamin B_{12} deficiency can be found in individuals with ileal Crohn's disease or after an ileal resection. Because the deficiency is not caused by a lack of dietary vitamin B_{12}, but rather from an inability to absorb vitamin B_{12}, oral supplementation with vitamin B_{12} tablets is not effective. In this setting, vitamin B_{12} must be given through a different route—as a monthly injection or a weekly application of nasal gel. Calcium and vitamin D deficiency are also commonly seen in Crohn's disease, both from reduced dietary intake and decreased absorption. These deficiencies usually can be treated with calcium and vitamin D tablets. If the vitamin D deficiency is severe, a prescription dose of a vitamin D tablet once to twice weekly for an average of 8 weeks can help to replace the body's stores before resuming a daily over-the-counter dose of vitamin D.

Zinc deficiency may also be found in Crohn's disease and should be supplemented with zinc tablets. Folic acid deficiency can occur in patients taking some medications that interfere with the normal absorption of folic acid; those patients should be on a daily folic acid supplement.

Iron deficiency is commonly found in Crohn's disease. Usually resulting from intestinal blood loss caused by an active flare of the disease, it can also be the result of reduced dietary intake and decreased absorption. In addition to treating the active Crohn's disease, patients are also often given an oral iron supplement. Patients who are unable to tolerate oral iron, which may cause gastrointestinal side effects, can be given intravenous iron instead. Magnesium deficiency as a result of intestinal losses can be seen in patients with chronic diarrhea and can be supplemented with magnesium oxide. Trace element deficiency is rare and is found only in individuals who have had extensive small bowel resection and those who are usually on home parenteral nutrition.

A common question is whether you should take any particular brand of vitamins given that many vitamins are marketed specifically for Crohn's disease or irritable bowel syndrome patients and are purported to be better than typical over-the-counter vitamins. The answer is no. The vitamins you can get in any drug store are usually equal to any of the more expensive vitamins that are marketed to specific patients. You need not spend more money on brand names when the generic vitamins are equally as good.

30. I'm chronically underweight. What can I do to gain weight?

Because of dietary restrictions, patients with Crohn's disease often find it difficult to maintain their ideal body weight. Whereas the majority of Americans are overweight and are constantly dieting, not infrequently individuals with Crohn's disease find themselves on the lower end of the scale trying to climb back up. There is no trick to gaining weight—eat more calories. However, when you have Crohn's disease, this is easier said than done. First, if you are underweight, you should take a daily multivitamin and be checked to see if you have any particular vitamin deficiencies that need to be corrected. Next, rather than trying to gorge yourself at breakfast, lunch, and dinner, which can leave you feeling overfilled, uncomfortable, and possibly with worsening symptoms, you should instead try eating small but frequent meals. The meals should consist of nutritional and high-caloric foods. Desserts and snacks in-between meals are encouraged. Although you should never force yourself to eat, you should also not deny yourself food whenever you are hungry. Last, if this is not enough to allow you to gain the desired amount of weight, nutritional supplements are often helpful. Many of these supplements do not contain lactose and are appropriate for those who may be lactose intolerant.

In addition to adding calories, moderate exercise with light weightlifting can also assist you in gaining weight. However, strenuous aerobic exercise can lead to further weight loss, so avoid this.

31. What foods should I eat or avoid if I have chronic diarrhea?

Diarrhea is an increase in stool volume or the frequency of bowel movements with excessive water content, occurring more than three times a day. Chronic diarrhea, defined as ongoing for more than three weeks, may be a sign of a serious problem. In addition to change in stool volume or frequency, patients with diarrhea may experience abdominal pain and bleeding with bowel movements.

Diarrhea is one of the most frustrating and embarrassing symptoms of Crohn's disease. Treating the underlying IBD is critical in managing chronic diarrhea; changes to your diet can also be helpful. Certain dietary substances are known to cause diarrhea. For instance, avoid eating foods with high fat content (such as foods that are greasy, fried, or very creamy). The fat in these foods works to speed up the contractions in your intestine that move digested food along. Caffeine, coffee, and tea also act as stimulants that can "rev up" the bowel and result in diarrhea. Fresh fruits and uncooked vegetables, high-fiber foods such as fiber-rich breads and cereals, and, at times, dairy products may also exacerbate diarrhea. Ice-cold liquids, even water, can cause cramps and diarrhea as well. In fact, too much of any type of liquid can lead to excess bowel movements. Glucose and electrolyte-based drinks, especially when diluted with water, are usually easier to absorb. Foods that may help solidify bowel movements include bananas, white bread, white rice, and cheese (if you're not lactose intolerant). See **Table 3** for a guide to what foods to eat and what foods to avoid.

TABLE 3 Foods to Include or Avoid with Chronic Diarrhea

Foods to avoid	Foods to include
High fat content (greasy, fried, creamy foods)	Bananas
Dairy products	White bread, white rice
Caffeine	Cheese
High-fiber foods	Boiled potatoes
Fresh fruit	Crackers, toast
Uncooked vegetables	Cooked carrots

Whether or not to add a fiber supplement for diarrhea can be confusing. As a general rule, high fiber of any kind is not a good idea during a flare. Those patients with Crohn's disease complicated by a perianal or rectovaginal fistula might have less leakage through the fistula if the stool can be made more solid with fiber. Your gastroenterologist and nutritionist can help you decide whether you might benefit from a fiber supplement.

32. What foods should I eat or avoid if I have a stricture?

When you have a stricture the intestine is narrowed, much like a pipe with a clog in it, which means certain foods may not pass through easily. Fortunately, because most food is digested and absorbed in the upper small bowel and most strictures in Crohn's disease occur in the lower small bowel, many patients do not know that they have a stricture. However, certain foods that are difficult to digest can travel undigested down through the intestinal tract and eventually block the stricture. Usually, this is a temporary situation, and you might experience abdominal pain and distention that lasts

DIET AND NUTRITION

anywhere from 30 minutes to a few hours shortly after you finish a meal. At other times, the blockage persists and you might experience severe abdominal pain, distention, vomiting, and inability to pass **flatus** (gas) or have a bowel movement. In these most severe cases, you need to be hospitalized for treatment.

Flatus

Gas passed per rectum.

You should avoid foods that are difficult to digest and, as a result, are more likely to cause a blockage. These include most fresh fruit and raw/uncooked vegetables, dried fruits, nuts, berries, corn and popcorn, and the less tender cuts of beef. As a rule of thumb, if what you are about to eat is very crunchy or requires a lot of chewing, you probably shouldn't eat it. Foods that are less fibrous are better to eat to avoid a blockage. These include fish, pasta, ground beef, small pieces of chicken, thoroughly cooked vegetables, rice, potatoes, eggs, cheese, most breads, most desserts, and soft fruits such as ripe bananas, applesauce, and melon. Each individual will have to learn which foods his or her body can tolerate and which foods he or she should avoid.

33. Is there a specific diet that I should follow if I have Crohn's disease?

Nutrition is an important part of everyday life. Good nutrition not only helps your body function at its best, but also promotes a strong immune system and a positive sense of well-being. This becomes more true for patients with Crohn's disease. Naturally, everyone should strive to eat a healthy, balanced diet, especially those who have Crohn's disease. This said, there is no specific diet you should follow, unless certain foods have made your symptoms worse.

The **specific carbohydrate diet** has been proposed by some as a good diet for patients with Crohn's disease. The specific carbohydrate diet is a grain-free, lactose-free, sucrose-free diet intended for patients with IBD and has also been suggested for patients with irritable bowel syndrome (IBS), celiac disease, and diverticulitis. The theory behind this diet is that carbohydrates (sugars) in a normal diet act as fuel for the overgrowth of bacteria and yeast in the small intestine. This overgrowth can cause an imbalance that damages the lining of the small intestine and impairs its ability to digest and absorb all nutrients, including carbohydrates. The excess of unabsorbed carbohydrates further fuels the cycle of overgrowth and imbalance. Promoters of this diet also believe that harmful toxins are produced by the excess bacteria and yeast inhabiting the small intestine.

By consuming only certain types of carbohydrates, people using this diet hope to eliminate bacterial and yeast overgrowth. Believers claim up to an 80% recovery rate in patients with Crohn's disease. Following are certain food guidelines for the specific carbohydrate diet.

Foods to avoid:

- Canned vegetables
- Canned fruits, unless they are packed in their own juices
- All grains, including flour, corn, oats, rye, rice, spelt, and soy
- Potatoes, yams, parsnips, chickpeas, bean sprouts, soybeans, mung beans, fava beans, and seaweed
- Processed meats, breaded or canned fish, processed cheeses, soft cheeses (ricotta, mozzarella), smoked or canned meat

Specific carbohydrate diet

A grain-free, lactose-free, sucrose-free diet that purportedly is beneficial in Crohn's disease and ulcerative colitis; a paucity of scientific evidence supports this claim.

DIET AND NUTRITION

- Milk or dried milk solids
- Buttermilk or acidophilus milk, commercially prepared yogurt and sour cream, soy milk, instant tea or coffee, coffee substitutes, and beer
- Cornstarch, arrowroot or other starches, chocolate or carob, bouillon cubes or instant soup bases, all products made with refined sugar, agar-agar, carrageenan or pectin, ketchup, ice cream, molasses, corn or maple syrup, flours made from legumes, baking powder, medication containing sugar, and all seeds

Foods to eat:

- Fresh and frozen vegetables and legumes (raw or cooked)
- Fresh, raw, or dried fruits
- Fresh or frozen meats, poultry, fish, and eggs
- Most nuts, including all-natural peanut butter
- Natural cheeses, homemade yogurt, and dry curd cottage cheese

Although this diet may seem like a simple, natural way to "treat" Crohn's disease, it has yet to be proved scientifically to help people with IBD. Although the "Foods to eat" list provides a healthy alternative to many items on the "Foods to avoid" list, several comments need to made about the diet as a whole. First and foremost, special diets should never be used as treatments for Crohn's disease and should never replace medications that have been proven to provide benefit. Although healthy diet choices should be a part of everyone's lifestyle, eliminating too many foods from a diet can be cumbersome. Patients who may also be lactose intolerant should avoid milk products. Certainly, fresh foods are a healthier alternative to canned or processed foods.

However, during a Crohn's flare, too many fresh fruits and vegetables can create a big fiber load for the small intestine and colon. While the specific carbohydrate diet is a reasonable nutrition plan with some modification, you should tell your gastroenterologist or nutritionist about this and any other special diets you may be considering. The bottom line is to beware of special diets that make big promises.

34. Do all patients with Crohn's disease have lactose intolerance?

Lactose intolerance is a very common problem for many people. It is caused by a deficiency of the lactase enzyme, which is found normally in the small intestine. Lactose is a major ingredient in dairy products such as milk, ice cream, yogurt, and cheese. There are also many less obvious sources of lactose. Did you know lactose can even be found in certain pills and deli meats? However, some nutritional supplements, even though they may look like a milkshake, do not contain lactose.

Symptoms of lactose intolerance include diarrhea, bloating, flatulence, and abdominal cramps after ingesting a lactose-containing product. Often, the higher fat content of milk products like ice cream can also contribute to these symptoms. The only treatments are lactose avoidance, taking supplemental lactase enzymes before eating or drinking a dairy product, or using products like milk/soy milk and ice cream that are specially made lactose-free. Remember that if you are lactose intolerant, you'll need to find other ways to supplement your calcium and vitamin D intake because you will no longer be getting them from your diet.

Because the lactase enzyme is found in the small intestine, individuals with Crohn's disease may also be prone to lactose intolerance as a result of inflammation and damage to the lining of the small intestine, which interfere with lactose absorption. Even healthy patients who get a "stomach bug" or viral gastroenteritis can have problems digesting lactose products for a little while until the lining of the bowels can heal. It is reasonable to eliminate dairy from your diet for a week or two after a diarrheal illness until the level of lactase enzyme can return to normal.

There are two ways to diagnose lactose intolerance. The most common way is to avoid dairy for 1 week and see if the cramps and diarrhea go away. Then drink a glass of milk and see if they recur. If you still are not sure whether you are lactose intolerant, your doctor can order a **lactose breath test** as a more objective measurement. Sugars (such as lactose) not absorbed properly in the small intestine make their way to the colon where they are metabolized by bacteria. These bacteria give off hydrogen, which quickly crosses the lining of the colon into the bloodstream and can be measured in the breath.

Lactose breath test

A test used to diagnose intolerance to lactose.

The day before the lactose breath test, you are instructed to avoid high-fiber foods that can cause an unusually high baseline level of hydrogen in the initial breath samples. Brushing your teeth also helps to decrease excess bacteria in your mouth that can also cause abnormally high baseline hydrogen readings. At the start of the test, you blow into the machine and the hydrogen level is measured. Then, you are instructed to drink a solution that has a high amount of lactose. Subsequent breath measurements for hydrogen are taken at 15- to 30-minute intervals over a 2-hour period. The total rise in hydrogen from the baseline measurement is then calculated. If this rise is greater than 20 parts per minute (ppm), lactose intolerance may be present. Certain situations such as recent antibiotic use, gastroenteritis, or small bowel bacterial overgrowth can cause the results to be inaccurate.

DIET AND NUTRITION

PART SIX

Related Conditions

Can Crohn's disease affect parts of my body other than just my bowels?

How can Crohn's disease affect my skin?

I often get little sores in my mouth, especially when my Crohn's disease is active. Are these related, and what can I do about them?

More . . .

35. Can Crohn's disease affect parts of my body other than just my bowels?

Crohn's disease can affect many different parts of your body (see **Table 4**). These are referred to as extraintestinal manifestations because these effects are found outside of the gastrointestinal tract. Extraintestinal manifestations are also called **systemic** symptoms because they reflect a process involving the body as a whole (a system), as opposed to local symptoms, which occur just in the intestinal tract. Systemic symptoms include fatigue, weight loss, anemia, and sometimes low-grade fevers. Extraintestinal manifestations can also be more localized to a specific organ. Organs that can be affected include the skin, eyes, joints, bones, kidneys, urinary tract, reproductive system, **gallbladder**, liver, and circulatory system. Although this list is quite long, extraintestinal manifestations do not occur in every patient.

Systemic

A process that involves the whole body, as opposed to a localized process; for example, fatigue is a systemic symptom, whereas lower back pain is a local symptom.

Gallbladder

A small sack adjacent to the liver where bile is stored.

TABLE 4 Extraintestinal Manifestations of Crohn's Disease

Common
Joint pain
Skin rashes
Mouth ulcers
Gallstones
Kidney stones
Anemia
Eye problems
Growth retardation in children
Uncommon
Liver disease (PSC)
Blood clots
Nerve damage
Lung disease
Pancreatitis (inflammation of the pancreas)
Pericarditis (inflammation around the heart)

Approximately 25% of individuals with Crohn's disease may develop one or more of the extraintestinal manifestations. Joint symptoms, such as arthritis, are the most common and are often seen together with skin and eye symptoms. Extraintestinal manifestations are found more often in individuals with Crohn's disease that primarily affects the colon; they are seen less often with predominantly small bowel disease.

We do not yet know what causes extraintestinal manifestations to develop, just as we do not know the cause of Crohn's disease. The leading theory is that because this disease is believed to be a result of a defect in the immune system, this same defect could potentially lead to inflammation in other areas of the body in addition to the gastrointestinal tract. Why certain people develop extraintestinal manifestations and others do not is still unknown.

The presence of extraintestinal manifestations often provides additional clues as to the level of activity of the underlying Crohn's disease. This is because, in many cases, extraintestinal manifestations often reflect ongoing intestinal inflammation that may not be apparent to either you or your gastroenterologist. In fact, some individuals use their extraintestinal manifestations as a signal as to when they are about to have a flare.

In general, effective treatment of the underlying disease usually leads to resolution of the extraintestinal symptoms. Some of the extraintestinal manifestations, however, run a course independent from the underlying Crohn's disease and do not improve along with improvements in the intestinal symptoms. It is also important to remember that systemic symptoms are sometimes a result of a drug-induced side effect and not from an extraintestinal manifestation.

Now you know why your gastroenterologist asks a long list of questions concerning many aspects of your overall health and does not focus just on your bowels at each visit. Crohn's disease involves not just the gastrointestinal tract, but can affect many different areas of the body as well. Indeed, at times the extraintestinal manifestations can be severe enough to overshadow a person's underlying intestinal symptoms. It is for this reason that you should inform your healthcare provider when you are having new symptoms, even if they seem unrelated to your bowel disease.

36. How can Crohn's disease affect my skin?

Erythema nodosum

A red, painful welling that can occur on the legs and arms in patients with IBD; can also be associated with other diseases.

Pyoderma gangrenosum

A skin ulcer that can occur in IBD patients anywhere on the skin, but most commonly is found on the extremities and immediately adjacent to a stoma.

The two most common types of skin rashes seen in individuals with Crohn's disease are **erythema nodosum** and **pyoderma gangrenosum**. Both rashes are very distinctive. Erythema nodosum appears as a painful, tender, reddish-purplish bump that occurs mostly on the shins; it can be found over the rest of the legs and arms as well. Erythema nodosum is a sign that your Crohn's disease is active. With treatment of the bowel disease, this rash should go away.

Unlike erythema nodosum, pyoderma gangrenosum can appear at any time and is not related to the activity of the underlying intestinal inflammation. Pyoderma gangrenosum is found most commonly on the legs and adjacent to an ileostomy or colostomy, although it can appear anywhere on your body. It starts as a red, inflamed area of skin usually smaller than the size of a dime. This inflamed area soon forms a punched-out, sharply demarcated ulcer with a raised reddish-purplish border. Pyoderma gangrenosum exhibits what is called the **pathergy phenomenon**. This is an unusual dermatologic condition in which a skin ulcer can get bigger and deeper as a result of even minor trauma, such as abrasive cleaning or pulling off a sticky dressing. For this reason, you should never attempt surgery on pyoderma gangrenosum. Because of the pathergy phenomenon, it can get large enough so that it takes months to heal. Pyoderma gangrenosum is not a common rash and, therefore, can be difficult to diagnose by the untrained eye. Any individual with Crohn's disease who develops an ulcer on the skin should be considered to have pyoderma gangrenosum until it is proved otherwise.

Pathergy phenomenon

An unusual dermatologic condition that occurs in pyoderma gangrenosum, in which even minor trauma can cause a skin ulcer to become bigger.

Several treatments are available for pyoderma gangrenosum. First and foremost, the ulcer should be bandaged with a nonstick dressing so as to avoid trauma when you change the dressing. First-line therapy usually consists of topical therapy with a corticosteroid ointment and cromolyn sodium. Topical cyclosporine has also shown good results. Corticosteroids can also be injected directly into the ulcer, but this approach is limited to use only on small ulcers and is not used as often as topical therapy. If topical therapy and/or corticosteroid injection is not successful, systemic therapy with oral or IV corticosteroids and various immune-modulating drugs has been found to be beneficial. In addition, even though pyoderma gangrenosum may occur in an individual whose Crohn's disease is in remission, it can also appear in someone with an active flare. In such a case, the active inflammation should be treated aggressively.

37. I often get little sores in my mouth, especially when my Crohn's disease is active. Are these related, and what can I do about them?

Sometimes Crohn's disease patients can develop small, painful sores in the mouth called **aphthous ulcers**. They can be very bothersome and appear much like canker sores. Infrequently, much larger ulcers can develop. Topical oral anesthetics can be helpful to numb the pain. A topical corticosteroid is often mixed in with the anesthetic. Usually the oral ulcers occur when the intestinal inflammation has become more active. Mouth sores can also develop as a side effect of some of the medications used to treat Crohn's disease. Antibiotics, for example, can cause **thrush**, which is an oral fungal infection. Also, the immune-modulating drugs can leave your body susceptible to viral infections such as the herpes simplex virus (HSV) or cytomegalovirus (CMV), both of which can cause sores on the lips and inside the mouth. Finally, Crohn's disease can directly affect the mouth. In these cases, the findings can range from multiple, small aphthous ulcers to large, irregular ulcers. Crohn's disease can also cause severe **gingivitis**. Last, **pyostomatitis vegetans** is a rare oral manifestation of Crohn's disease. Often considered to be an oral presentation of pyoderma gangrenosum, multiple small pustules, ulcers, and abscesses occur in the oral cavity.

Aphthous ulcers

Small ulcers that can occur in Crohn's disease or ulcerative colitis.

Thrush

Oral (mouth and throat) fungal infection; appears as a whitish plaque on the tongue and on the inside lining of the mouth.

Gingivitis

Inflammation of the gums.

Pyostomatitis vegetans

A rare form of Crohn's disease in which multiple, small pustules, ulcers, and abscesses develop in the oral cavity.

38. My joints are often stiff and sore. Is this related to my Crohn's disease?

Individuals with Crohn's disease often complain of having sore and stiff joints. The medical term for soreness and stiffness in the joints is arthralgia. Arthritis is when the joints are actually inflamed—painful, red, swollen, and warm. These joint symptoms can be divided into two categories: those that affect the central or spinal joints (back, pelvis, hips), and those that affect the peripheral joints (shoulders, elbows, wrists, fingers, knees, ankles, toes).

Peripheral arthralgias may be seen in up to 30% of individuals with Crohn's disease. These patients often experience painful, stiff joints throughout their body. A single joint or several joints can be affected at the same time, or the pain can migrate from one joint to another. Sometimes a true arthritis can be seen with a red, hot, and swollen joint. Arthritis associated with Crohn's disease is different from both **osteoarthritis** (so-called wear-and-tear arthritis) and rheumatoid arthritis. The type of arthritis associated with Crohn's disease is a nondestructive form of arthritis, meaning that it does not permanently damage the joints. This is different from osteoarthritis and rheumatoid arthritis that do lead to joint destruction.

For this reason, it is important for your healthcare provider to investigate any new joint symptoms you have, because they may be caused by a variety of illnesses. If a single joint is red, hot, or swollen, it could mean the joint is infected. **Gout** is another condition that can cause pain in a single joint, often the big toe. In gout, uric acid crystals form and become concentrated in the joint fluid, causing inflammation and pain. Your healthcare provider may want to remove a sample of fluid from the joint with a small needle to send for laboratory analysis and examination under a microscope to rule out these other causes of joint pain.

Osteoarthritis

Arthritis caused by natural wear and tear on the joints; commonly occurs in older individuals, but can also be found in younger athletes as a result of years of trauma.

Gout

Type of arthritis characterized by uric acid crystal deposition in the joints; often presents as a red, swollen, painful big toe.

Peripheral arthralgias associated with Crohn's disease usually mirror the activity of the underlying bowel disease. In other words, the joint pains often develop as a result of an active flare, sometimes just before a flare is about to happen. Accordingly, treatment of underlying bowel symptoms usually makes the joint pains feel better.

Central (spinal) arthralgias occur in approximately 5% of people with Crohn's disease. The joints that are most affected include those of the lower spine and pelvis, specifically the sacroiliac joints within the pelvis. Patients may develop pain or stiffness in the lower back that is worse in the morning upon waking and improves with activity throughout the day. Unlike peripheral arthralgias, arthritis affecting the central joints can lead to permanent damage, when joints fuse together in the vertebral column, as well as in the sacroiliac region. Central arthritis is also different from peripheral arthralgias in that it is not necessarily associated with the level of bowel activity. In fact, central arthritis can show up years before bowel symptoms occur. Treatment of bowel symptoms does not help this type of arthritis. Rather, treatment is targeted toward helping control the arthritis symptoms. Range of motion exercises, physical therapy, and moist heat applied to the back can be helpful.

39. Is it true that Crohn's disease can also affect my eyes?

Eye disorders associated with Crohn's disease are among the most serious of the extraintestinal manifestations. Left untreated, they can result in permanent damage, including scarring and blindness. It is for this reason that you and your healthcare provider should be quick to consult an ophthalmologist for prompt diagnosis and treatment of any eye symptoms (as discussed here). The ophthalmologist will use a slit lamp test (a microscopic view of the inside structures of the eye) to detect different abnormalities. Usually, treatment of the underlying bowel disease can help alleviate the **ocular** symptoms. Sometimes corticosteroid eye drops are used as well. Regardless, any new eye symptoms must be evaluated promptly because delay in treatment can cause lasting damage to the eyes.

Ocular
Refers to the eye.

Episcleritis
Inflammation of the whites of the eye.

Iritis
Inflammation of the iris, which is the colored part of the eye.

Uveitis
Inflammation of the uvea, which is the central part of the eye (the iris is part of the uvea).

The three most common eye disorders associated with Crohn's disease are **episcleritis**, **iritis**, and **uveitis**. These names correspond to different structures in the eye that have become inflamed. Episcleritis refers to inflammation of the white of the eye; iritis refers to inflammation of the colored part of the eye; and uveitis refers to inflammation of the central portion of the eye. Often, the tiny blood vessels of the eye become inflamed, causing them to dilate or expand, which is what causes the eye to become red. Other symptoms include pain, sensitivity to light, and blurred vision. These ocular disorders often occur along with arthritis and erythema nodosum. Usually the problem will affect only one eye at a time. You should contact your gastroenterologist immediately to be evaluated. Often the ophthalmologist will prescribe steroid drops to alleviate the inflammation and prevent any damage to the eye.

Other problems that affect the eyes, such as cataracts and **glaucoma**, can be side effects of the long-term use of corticosteroids. Needing reading glasses as you get older, on the other hand, has nothing to do with Crohn's disease—it's simply part of the natural aging process.

Glaucoma
Increased pressure within the eye.

40. How does Crohn's disease cause you to become anemic?

Anemia is a condition that occurs when the body is depleted of red blood cells. The two main causes of anemia are loss of blood and decreased production of red blood cells. Blood loss is most commonly caused by gastrointestinal bleeding. Rapid gastrointestinal bleeding is uncommon in Crohn's disease and suggests that there is another potential source, such as a bleeding ulcer or bleeding from diverticulosis. Chronic, or slow, blood loss causing iron deficiency anemia is commonly seen in Crohn's disease. A variety of illnesses can cause anemia from decreased production of red blood cells, including iron and vitamin deficiencies, lead poisoning, bone marrow problems, chronic kidney failure, and certain blood disorders such as **sickle cell anemia** and **thalassemia**. Some medications may also cause anemia. Caveat: Anyone over the age of 50 who develops new-onset iron deficiency anemia should be checked thoroughly for an underlying gastrointestinal cancer such as colon cancer as a possible cause.

Individuals with Crohn's disease involving the small bowel can develop anemia for several reasons. To start with, inflammation or subsequent surgical removal of the small bowel can cause malabsorption that leads to inadequate uptake of vitamins and nutrients. Bodily stores of iron, vitamin B_{12}, and folate can become depleted, leading to anemia. Also, commonly used medications in Crohn's disease can cause anemia; the anemia can sometimes be severe enough to warrant stopping the medication. Last, active Crohn's disease can lead to anemia of chronic disease as a result of stress on the body as a whole.

Sickle cell anemia

An inherited blood disorder that can cause anemia.

Thalassemia

An inherited blood disorder that can cause anemia.

Symptoms of chronic anemia include tiredness, pale skin, shortness of breath on exertion, and decreased exercise capacity. This happens because red blood cells deliver oxygen to the various tissues and organs of the body. As the number of red blood cells decreases in anemia, the body does not get enough oxygen to work at full capacity. If you have underlying heart disease, chest pain and shortness of breath can be important signals that your heart is under excessive stress and that the anemia needs to be corrected immediately with a blood transfusion. Severe anemia can lead to a rapid pulse, decrease in blood pressure, and episodes of passing out. When this occurs, an immediate blood transfusion is usually needed. However, the majority of Crohn's disease patients with chronic anemia do not need blood transfusions, but usually get better with folate, B_{12}, or iron supplementation. Bleeding from ulcerative colitis does not usually cause significant anemia and is rarely severe enough to require a blood transfusion.

PART SEVEN

Other Questions and Concerns

Is it safe to have a baby if I have Crohn's disease?

Can Crohn's disease affect fertility in men?

Can I take Crohn's disease medications while I am breastfeeding?

More . . .

41. Is it safe to have a baby if I have Crohn's disease?

Yes, it is safe to have a baby if you have Crohn's disease. This disease most commonly affects young men and women during their childbearing years, so naturally many individuals with Crohn's disease are concerned about whether they can safely have children. Pregnancy itself does not appear to pose any increased risk to women who have Crohn's disease as compared to those who do not. However, studies have shown that women who have active, poorly controlled Crohn's disease during pregnancy are more at risk for miscarriage, premature delivery, and stillbirth. For women whose disease is in remission, there is still a small risk for premature delivery and low birth weight. That being said, women with Crohn's disease in remission generally have normal pregnancies and deliver healthy babies. It is important to note, however, that even for the average healthy woman without Crohn's disease there is still a 2% to 3% chance of having a complication during pregnancy. In other words, although it is safe to have a baby if you have Crohn's disease in remission, there is still some degree of risk inherent in any pregnancy. Emerging research regarding biologic medications taken during pregnancy has shown that these medications can cross the placenta, and elevated drug levels have been detected in newborns. While we do not believe this necessarily creates a harmful situation, some healthcare providers are recommending that live newborn vaccines be delayed.

42. Can Crohn's disease affect fertility in men?

Crohn's disease generally does not cause fertility problems in men. However, it is possible that one of the drugs commonly used to treat Crohn's disease can cause decreased sperm count, reduced sperm motility, and abnormal sperm shape. If you are taking any medication for Crohn's disease, check with your healthcare provider about its effect on fertility. It is likely that another effective medication can be substituted. Men who have had pelvic surgery may have a low risk of infertility and choose to bank their sperm beforehand.

43. Can I take Crohn's disease medications while I am breastfeeding?

Many of the medications listed as safe during pregnancy are also considered safe for use during breastfeeding. There are some medications that are not recommended for breastfeeding mothers—ask your healthcare provider which ones these are. This can be a very emotional issue for some women and should be discussed at length either prior to or early on in the pregnancy. It is important to remember that if you have a flare, you may become too ill to breastfeed. So, although you may prefer to breastfeed and should be allowed to if you can, bottle-feeding may be the safest option if the alternative is a Crohn's disease flare in a new mother.

44. If I have Crohn's disease, what is the chance that my children will have it?

If you have Crohn's disease, there is about a 4% to 9% chance that you will have a child with it. If both parents have Crohn's disease, the risk for the child increases to 36%. However this risk is small, and just because you have Crohn's disease doesn't automatically mean that your kids will have it, too.

Several genes have been identified as associated with Crohn's disease. One is called the NOD2/CARD 15 gene, which has more than 60 variations. For example, three of these NOD2/CARD 15 gene variations have been identified in 27% of people with Crohn's disease specifically involving the ileum. It is important to remember, though, that although these genes are involved in Crohn's disease, they are only part of the story. The NOD2/ CARD 15 gene is believed to play the role of a permissive gene, meaning that the gene cannot cause the disease by itself, but can help facilitate the expression of Crohn's disease. In other words, even if you carry one of these genes, you will not automatically develop Crohn's disease. Rather, Crohn's disease may be caused by a combination of genetic influences and an environmental trigger, such as a bacterium.

45. Does stress affect Crohn's disease?

Based on scientific evidence, the following statements can be made:

1. Emotional stress alone cannot cause a person to develop Crohn's disease.
2. Emotional stress alone cannot induce a flare of Crohn's disease.
3. There is a no higher incidence of major psychiatric illness in patients with Crohn's disease than the general population.

That being said, many people with Crohn's disease still believe that major life stressors coincide with a flare. Certainly stress can make it harder to deal with Crohn's disease when it is flaring. Additionally, patients with Crohn's disease, or any chronic illness, who also suffer from depression, have a more difficult clinical course than a chronically ill patient without depression. In addition, some of the corticosteroids that are used to treat Crohn's disease may cause severe mood swings, irritability/anger, tremulousness, insomnia, and depression.

Individuals under stress with or without a history of Crohn's disease commonly suffer gastrointestinal symptoms such as cramps, bloating, constipation, and/or diarrhea. This is similar to getting a headache due to stress. If these symptoms occur frequently and in certain patterns, they are likely due to irritable bowel syndrome, or IBS. The body often senses and reacts to changes in environment long before our conscious mind registers them. Unfortunately, those with Crohn's disease often have IBS, too. IBS symptoms, such as the ones mentioned here, can often occur despite the fact that the Crohn's disease is in remission. Additional strategies can be used to help with IBS symptoms.

PART EIGHT

Communicating with Your Gastroenterologist

What should I discuss with my gastroenterologist?

How often should I see my gastroenterologist?

What should I do about new problems and questions?

More . . .

46. What should I discuss with my gastroenterologist?

Open, honest communication is the key to a true partnership with your gastroenterologist. In fact, research has shown that successful communication between a patient and a clinician can lead to better patient outcomes (e.g., better emotional health, better symptom resolution, better functional and physical status). For your gastroenterologist to provide the best possible care for you, he or she needs to know more than the facts of your illness. In order to decide what treatment is best for you, her or she may look at your particular case, you personally, your generally philosophy about your health, and your ability to cope with illness.

Should I keep a daily journal?

Keeping a daily journal is a good idea, as it allows you to track your symptoms and provides you and your gastroenterologist with information about the course of your disease. If you are taking medication, a daily journal may show whether or not the medication has taken effect. People with Crohn's disease are encouraged to track the number and quality of daily bowel movements (bloody, firm, etc.), weight loss, severity of gastrointestinal inflammation/cramping, diet, nausea/vomiting, and level of stress. While neither stress nor diet can cause Crohn's disease or even cause a flare, both diet and stress can exacerbate symptoms that are already present.

What types of medications are used to treat Crohn's disease?

Several types of medications are used to treat patients with Crohn's disease. The major types include the **aminosalicylates (5-ASA) drugs**, **immune-modulating drugs**, corticosteroids, antibiotics, and **biologic agents**.

Aminosalicylates: The 5-ASA (aminosalicylates) drugs are usually taken orally and act to reduce inflammation, but they do not affect the immune system. In addition to oral preparations, other 5-ASA treatments include **retention enemas** and **suppositories**.

Corticosteroids: Corticosteroids are potent anti-inflammatory drugs and are used in oral, rectal, and intravenous (IV) forms. Corticosteroids reduce the inflammation associated with Crohn's disease. Although very effective for short-term use, corticosteroids have limited effectiveness for long-term use and are associated with a number of side-effects and complications.

Immune modulating drugs: Immune modulating drugs (also known as immunomodulators) are used in patients who do not respond to anti-inflammatory medications, such as aminosalicylates and corticosteroids. These types of drugs work by modulating/suppressing the body's immune system to prevent the inflammation associated with Crohn's disease. By suppressing the immune system, one of the potential complications of immune modulating drugs is an increase in the risk of infections. Patients on immunomodulators need regular monitoring of their blood to look for decreased red and white blood cells, as well as elevation in the liver function tests (which are possible side effects of the medications). Individuals on these types of medications should

5-ASAs

Aminosalicylates are medications used to treat the inflammation associated with inflammatory bowel disease; they come in oral and topical forms.

Immunomodulators

A class of drugs that modulates or suppresses the immune system.

Biologic agents

A group of therapeutic medications that include monoclonal antibodies.

Retention enema

A process of instilling liquid (usually oil based) into the rectum, where it is retained for several hours, to soften stool.

Suppository

A small plug of medicine, often cylindrical, that is inserted into the vagina or anus, and is designed to melt at body temperature.

also contact their healthcare provider at the first signs of an infection.

Biologic agents: Biologic agents are drugs that target specific proteins in the body. Some biologic agents block the production of TNF. TNF is a protein that circulates in the blood and is associated with inflammation in the intestines. Another class of biologic agents targets the **adhesion molecules** that allow white blood cells to stick to the wall of the intestines.

Antibiotics: Antibiotics are also used to treat Crohn's disease, as well as infectious complications of this disease, such as an abscess. Antibiotics are also commonly used to treat fistulas and abscesses around the anus, which may be seen in individuals with Crohn's disease.

Antispasmodics: In some situations, agents that help reduce the spasms of pain and the bouts of diarrhea are used in combination with the above medications to treat the symptoms of abdominal cramps and frequent loose stools.

Prebiotics/Probiotics: Many individuals have started using **prebiotics** and **probiotics** to treat IBD. Prebiotics are nondigestible nutrients that help promote the growth of "good" bacteria in your body. Probiotics are the actual "good" bacteria themselves in the form of a dietary supplement. While this may be a compelling idea and sound good, there is little data supporting the use of prebiotics and probiotics.

Elemental diet: A liquid diet of predigested nutrients, called an elemental diet, has been successfully used to treat children with Crohn's disease. In this case, no regular food is allowed, with all nutrition derived from

Adhesion molecules

Proteins located on the surface of a white blood cell that help it stick to the lining of the intestines.

Prebiotics

Nondigestible food ingredients that are ingested by the normal bacteria occurring in the colon. They are believed to aid in digestion.

Probiotics

Healthy bacteria that can be ingested with the goal of repopulating the digestive system with "good" bacteria.

the **elemental diet**. As most individuals find that an elemental diet tastes bad, placement of a feeding tube is required to administer the liquid diet. Newer formulations taste better and may not require a feeding tube.

Pain relief: Acetaminophen is the preferred pain medication for use in patients with Crohn's disease. You should not use narcotic medications chronically, given the potential for addiction. Patients with chronic pain unrelated to active Crohn's disease might benefit from a referral to a comprehensive pain center.

Prophylactic therapy: Crohn's disease can recur after surgery, so medications may be started soon after surgery in individuals at high risk for recurrent Crohn's disease in an effort to decrease the chance that the disease will return. Close follow-up with a gastroenterologist is important after surgery.

Will I need surgery?

Although Crohn's disease is usually adequately treated with medical therapy, approximately 70% to 80% of patients will still need to undergo surgery at some point in their lifetime. Surgery becomes necessary when medical treatment is no longer able to keep the symptoms of Crohn's disease under control, or when a complication arises.

When a person's Crohn's disease is no longer responsive to medical therapy, the decision to perform surgery should be made jointly by you, your gastroenterologist, and your surgeon. To achieve the best outcome, all three parties should be in agreement. Often, you may want surgery because you are frustrated by your ill-

Elemental diet

A regulated intake of liquid nutrients that includes fats, sugars, amino acids, vitamins, and minerals.

ness and feel that you won't get better. However, your physicians may encourage you to be patient, knowing from experience and extensive training that the medicine might need more time to work fully. In addition, because Crohn's disease has such a high postoperative recurrence rate, physicians are often reluctant to recommend surgery until all reasonable medical options have been exhausted. At other times, however, a physician may recommend surgery knowing that there are no good medical options left, while you may not yet be ready psychologically for an operation.

One of the many factors that physicians take into account when deciding on surgery is whether you are on any medication that either has caused or has the potential to cause you harm.

When a complication occurs, the decision to have surgery is more clear-cut. If a bowel perforation, bowel obstruction, toxic megacolon, sepsis, or an abscess develops, surgery is almost always indicated. This is not to say that nonoperative therapy might not be attempted, but that the threshold to operate is much lower and the decision is usually made much quicker.

Should I get a second opinion?

Most patients with Crohn's disease have a mild form of the disease that can easily be managed by a general gastroenterologist; however, some individuals have a more aggressive form of the disease. In particular, patients with extensive Crohn's disease and ongoing symptoms, despite the use of steroids or immunomodulators, are at increased risk for complications and might benefit from a second opinion.

Keep in mind that your gastroenterologist wants you to get better and wants you to take an active role in your ongoing care. Don't be embarrassed to ask for a second opinion about treatment options, prognosis, or any aspect of your healthcare plan—it does not mean you don't trust your gastroenterologist, it just means you want to learn more about your disease. You may be surprised to find that some insurance companies recommend or encourage patients to get second opinions. Some people choose to consult with a second gastroenterologist when:

- They are considering surgery
- Their clinician prescribes a new medication
- They are not seeing an improvement in symptoms despite repeated visits to their gastroenterologist
- They want to learn more about alternative treatments

There are multiple places to look when you are researching gastroenterologists' credentials to find one to consult for a second opinion. Hospital websites list faculty members and their credentials, health insurance companies have lists of resources in your community, and even your gastroenterologist can suggest other clinicians for you to see. Another resource is the Crohn's and Colitis Foundation of America, which provides a list of gastroenterologists with expertise in treating IBD.

Ask your clinician to send your medical records to the gastroenterologist that will be providing a second opinion. If you will be bringing the records with you, it will be helpful to have notes from office visits, results from colonoscopies, and pathology reports. Also, for reference, plan to bring along original biopsy slides, X-rays,

CT scans, and MRI scans. Ask the gastroenterologist prior to your appointment, as they may be able to provide you with a list of items they would like you to bring.

47. How often should I see my gastroenterologist?

You and your gastroenterologist will work to develop your treatment plan, which will include how often to schedule appointments. Certainly contact his or her office if new problems arise, or keep a list of questions and concerns to bring to the next visit.

48. What should I do about new problems and questions?

While you should write down all problems and questions to discuss with your healthcare provider, you should try to focus on the new problems and limit your questions to the most important ones. Written descriptions and your own opinion of the diagnosis will suggest other questions by the clinician. Write down the name or diagnosis of the problem.

It may also improve your understanding if you ask to have everything explained in lay (nonmedical) terms. Be certain you fully understand your diagnosis. Ask your gastroenterologist's office if they have printed information on the new subject to give you and ask what the procedure is to get results of testing and consultations. For example, there may be a special telephone number to call to get results.

49. Will I be given a treatment plan?

You and your gastroenterologist should create a treatment plan together. After you and your provider have developed the treatment plan, follow it closely. And be honest—do not say you will follow the treatment plan if you will not (e.g., avoiding caffeine). Furthermore, be sure the treatment plan takes into account your lifestyle, religious, and cultural preferences. Make sure you know which follow-up steps to take, when to call and why, and with whom you should speak (e.g., provider, receptionist, nurse). If you notice problems or side effects, notify your gastroenterologist immediately. If you wish to change methods of treatment, then express this to your gastroenterologist. You need to be a partner in developing the treatment plan.

50. Where can I find a support network?

There are many resources available for people diagnosed with Crohn's disease. A list of useful organizations and their contact information is show in **Table 5**. The Crohn's and Colitis Foundation of America (CCFA) has an information resource center that provides accurate and current disease-related information. There are local CCFA chapters throughout the country that run educational programs as well as support groups. You can find a support group near you by searching the CCFA website or calling their toll-free number. There are also a few online support groups available. The websites www.dailystrength.org and www.supportgroups.com both have dedicated Crohn's disease online support groups. The website www.crohnsforum.com is a site solely for online support targeted to those living with or affected by Crohn's disease.

TABLE 5 Resources on Crohn's Disease

Name of Organization	Web site	Phone number
American College of Gastroenterology	http://www.acg.gi.org	301-263-9000
American Gastroentero-logical Association	http://www.gastro.org	301-654-2055
Crohn's and Colitis Foundation of America	http://www.ccfa.org	800-932-2423
IBS Support Foundation	http://www.IBDSF.com	323-938-8090
HealthCentral	http://www.healthcentral.com/ibd/	703-302-1040
National Digestive Diseases Information Clearinghouse	http://digestive.niddk.nih.gov	800-891-5389
Reach Out for Youth	http://www.reachoutforyouth.org	631-293-3102
The Foundation for Clinical Research in IBD	http://www.MyIBD.org	
UC and Crohn's: A Site for Teens	http://www.ucandcrohns.org	
United Ostomy Association of America	http://www.ostomy.org	800-826-0826

Glossary

5-ASAs: Aminosalicylates are medications used to treat the inflammation associated with inflammatory bowel disease; they come in oral and topical forms.

Abdominal cavity: The part of the body below the chest and above the pelvic bone that contains the internal organs, including the small intestine, colon, stomach, liver, pancreas, kidneys, and bladder.

Abdominal X-ray: A radiologic examination that provides an image of structures and organs in the abdomen—helpful in detecting a bowel obstruction or perforation.

Abscess: A walled-off collection of pus; in Crohn's disease, an abscess is most commonly found around the anus or rectum, but can occur anywhere in the body.

Adhesion: Scar tissue that forms internally, usually after an operation; a common cause of bowel obstruction.

Adhesion molecules: Proteins located on the surface of a white blood cell that help it stick to the lining of the intestines.

Aminosalicylate: A class of drugs used in Crohn's disease.

Anastomosis: A surgically made connection between two structures in the body; in Crohn's disease, this is usually between two segments of intestine after a resection, or between the intestine and the skin to create an ileostomy or colostomy.

Anemia: A lower-than-normal number of red blood cells.

Angiography: A radiologic test that looks at the blood vessels.

Anorexia: An eating disorder in which someone does not want to eat.

Anoscopy: A procedure in which a rigid, short, straight, lighted tube is used to examine the anal canal; usually performed on a special tilt table that positions the patient with the head down and buttocks up. An excellent test to examine for an anal fissure or hemorrhoids.

Antineutrophil cytoplasmic antibody (ANCA): An antibody found in the blood that is associated with the presence of ulcerative colitis.

Anti-Saccharomyces cerevisiae antibody (ASCA): An antibody found in the blood that is associated with the presence of Crohn's disease.

Anus: The outside opening of the rectum.

Aphthous ulcers: Small ulcers that can occur in Crohn's disease or ulcerative colitis.

Arthritis: Inflammation of the joints; individuals with arthritis often have pain, redness, tenderness, and swelling in the affected joints.

Autoimmune: An inflammatory process in which your immune system attacks part of your own body, such as the colon in ulcerative colitis.

Bacterial overgrowth: A condition in which an overgrowth of normal intestinal flora occurs; usually seen in the setting of an intestinal stricture.

Barium: Barium sulfate, when mixed with water, becomes a white chalky substance that is ingested and allows radiologic examination of the rectum, colon, or small intestine.

Barium enema: A radiologic examination of the rectum and colon performed by instilling barium through the rectum and taking X-rays as it travels through the colon; an excellent test to detect strictures, inflammation, and fistulas in the colon.

Biologic agents: A group of therapeutic medications that include monoclonal antibodies.

Biopsy: Usually performed during an endoscopy, a small piece of mucosa (inside lining of the intestine) is removed and examined under a microscope; an excellent test to characterize types of inflammation and detect dysplasia and cancer.

Bowel: Another name for intestine; that is, small intestine means the same as small bowel.

Bypass: An operation in which a segment of diseased intestine is bypassed by connecting the healthy intestine above the diseased segment to the healthy intestine below.

Cancer: An uncontrolled growth of cells in the body that can form a tumor and can spread, or metastasize, to other areas of the body.

Capsule endoscopy: A test in which the patient swallows a large pill containing a camera and wears a sensor device on the abdomen; the capsule passes naturally through the small intestine while transmitting video images to the sensor, which stores data that can be downloaded to a computer.

CCFA: Crohn's and Colitis Foundation of America.

Cecum: The first part of the large intestine; a pouch-like area into which the ileum opens.

Cell: The smallest unit in the body; millions of cells attached together make up the organs and tissues.

Cholangitis: Infection of the bile ducts; can occur in primary sclerosing cholangitis (PSC).

Colonic transit time: The time it takes for stool to travel from the beginning of the colon (the cecum) to the rectum.

Colonoscopy: An endoscopic procedure in which a small, thin, flexible lighted tube with a camera on the end is passed through the rectum into the colon and, at times, into the ileum; an excellent test to detect inflammation and strictures in the rectum, colon, and ileum, and one that allows for a biopsy to be taken.

Colostomy: Surgically created connection between the colon and skin to allow for the diversion of fecal material; the waste empties into a bag attached to the skin.

Corticosteroid: A potent anti-inflammatory drug.

Crohn's colitis: Crohn's disease of the colon.

Crohn's disease: An intestinal disease characterized by chronic intestinal inflammation; can affect any area of the gastrointestinal tract.

Distention: Abdominal bloating usually from excess amounts of gas in the intestines; can be a sign of a bowel obstruction.

Duodenum: The first part of the small intestine just beyond the stomach.

Dysplasia: A premalignant cellular change seen on biopsy prior to the development of cancer; can occur in the colon in Crohn's colitis, but can also be found in other organs not related to IBD, such as cervical dysplasia (which is what a Pap smear examines for) or esophageal dysplasia in Barrett's esophagus.

Elemental diet: A regulated intake of liquid nutrients that includes fats, sugars, amino acids, vitamins, and minerals.

Episcleritis: Inflammation of the whites of the eye.

ERCP: Endoscopic retrograde cholangiopancreatography; this is an endoscopic procedure used to examine the bile duct and the pancreatic duct. This procedure is performed for a variety of reasons, including detecting and removing stones in the common bile duct, to detect tumors involving the bile or pancreatic ducts, and to diagnose primary sclerosing cholangitis.

Erythema nodosum: A red, painful welling that can occur on the legs and arms in patients with IBD.

Evaluation under anesthesia (EUA): Physical examination of the rectum and perirectal area performed when the patient is anesthetized; usually done to evaluate for an abscess and/or fistula.

Extraintestinal manifestations: Signs of IBD that are found outside of the gastrointestinal tract, hence the term extraintestinal.

Fistula: A tunnel connecting two structures that are not normally connected; examples include a fistula between the rectum and vagina (rectovaginal fistula) or the colon and bladder (colovesicular fistula).

Flatus: Gas passed per rectum.

Food allergy: An immune system response to a food that the body mistakenly believes is harmful.

Food intolerance: An adverse reaction to food that does not involve the immune system.

Gallbladder: A small sack adjacent to the liver where bile is stored.

Gallstones: Stones that form in the gallbladder.

Gastroenterologist: A physician who specializes in diseases of the gastrointestinal tract, liver, and pancreas.

Gastrointestinal tract: The digestive tube that starts at the mouth and ends at the anus.

Genetic predisposition: An inherited trait that makes one more likely to develop a disease.

Gingivitis: Inflammation of the gums.

Glaucoma: Increased pressure within the eye.

Gout: Type of arthritis characterized by uric acid crystal deposition in the joints; often presents as a red, swollen, painful big toe.

Granuloma: A certain type of cell found in Crohn's disease; can also be seen in other, nongastrointestinal diseases.

Granulomatous colitis: Crohn's disease of the colon.

Granulomatous enteritis: Crohn's disease of the small bowel.

Ileum: Lowest section of the small intestine.

Immune dysregulation: Failure of the body to appropriately regulate the immune system; this lack of regulation is believed to be integral to the development of Crohn's disease and ulcerative colitis.

Immunomodulator: A class of drugs that modulates or suppresses the immune system.

Immune system: An internal network of organs, cells, and structures that work to guard your body against foreign substances, such as infections.

Inflammation: A process characterized by swelling, warmth, redness, and/or tenderness; can occur in any organ.

Iritis: Inflammation of the iris, which is the colored part of the eye.

Irritable bowel syndrome (IBS): A functional disorder characterized by atypical abdominal pain, diarrhea, constipation, diarrhea alternating with constipation, the feeling of incomplete fecal evacuation, or any combination of these symptoms.

Kidney stones: Stones that form in the kidneys.

Lactase: The intestinal enzyme responsible for the breakdown of lactose; deficiency in this enzyme leads to lactose malabsorption.

Lactose breath test: A test used to diagnose intolerance to lactose.

Lactose intolerance: The inability to absorb dairy products caused by a deficiency of the lactase enzyme; a type of malabsorption disorder.

Malabsorption: A condition in which the small intestine is not able to absorb nutrients and vitamins.

Malnutrition: A condition in which your body has not taken in enough nutrients and vitamins to maintain good health.

MRI: Magnetic resonance imaging; a radiologic examination that uses a magnetic field to create a detailed picture of structures and organs within the body. An MRI is especially helpful in detecting abdominal and pelvic abscesses.

Mucosa: The innermost lining of the intestines.

Nasogastric tube: A long, flexible tube that is passed through the nose into the stomach and is used to suction out the stomach in the setting of a bowel obstruction or sometimes after an operation.

Obstruction: A blockage of the small intestine or colon.

Ocular: Refers to the eye.

Osteoarthritis: Arthritis caused by natural wear and tear on the joints; commonly occurs in older individuals, but can also be found in younger athletes as a result of years of trauma.

Osteoporosis: A severe decrease in bone density; can occur after long-term use of corticosteroids.

Pathergy phenomenon: An unusual dermatologic condition that occurs in pyoderma gangrenosum, in which even minor trauma can cause a skin ulcer to become bigger.

Pathologist: A physician trained in the evaluation of organs, tissues, and cells, usually under a microscope; assists in determining and characterizing the presence of disease.

Perforation: A rupture or abnormal opening of the intestine that allows intestinal contents to escape into the abdominal cavity.

Perianal: The area adjacent to the outside of the anus; common site for abscess and fistula formation.

Prebiotics: Nondigestible food ingredients that are ingested by the normal bacteria occurring in the colon. They are believed to aid in digestion.

Prevalence: The number of people affected by a disease in a population at a specific time.

Probiotics: Healthy bacteria that can be ingested with the goal of re-populating the digestive system with "good" bacteria.

Proctoscopy: A procedure in which a rigid, straight, lighted tube is used to examine the rectum; usually this examination is performed on a special tilt table that positions the patient with the head down and buttocks up. Although this procedure has mostly been replaced by flexible sigmoid-oscopy, it is still an excellent test to examine the rectum.

Pyoderma gangrenosum: A skin ulcer that can occur in IBD patients anywhere on the skin, but most commonly is found on the extremities and immediately adjacent to a stoma.

Pyostomatitis vegetans: A rare form of Crohn's disease in which multiple, small pustules, ulcers, and abscesses develop in the oral cavity.

Recurrence: The reappearance of a disease.

Remission: The state of having no active disease. It can refer to clinical remission, meaning no symptoms are present; endoscopic remission, meaning no disease is detected endoscopically; or histologic remission, meaning no active inflammation is detected on biopsy.

Retention enema: A process of instilling liquid (usually oil based) into the rectum, where it is retained for several hours, to soften stool.

Risk: The chance or probability that something will or will not happen.

Sedation: Also called conscious sedation, or moderate sedation; sedation is a form of moderate anesthesia in which the patient is given medication to induce a state of relaxation. Patients under sedation are sleepy and are less likely to feel discomfort.

Seton: A small, thin, flexible piece of tubing that is inserted through the skin, into an abscess, out of the abscess, into the rectum, and then out through the anus where the two ends are tied together.

Short gut syndrome: A condition of severe malabsorption caused by extensive small bowel resection.

Sickle cell anemia: An inherited blood disorder that can cause anemia.

Sigmoidoscopy: This procedure is basically a "short" colonoscopy and is used to examine the rectum and left colon.

Specific carbohydrate diet: A grain-free, lactose-free, sucrose-free diet that purportedly is beneficial in Crohn's disease and ulcerative colitis; a paucity of scientific evidence supports this claim.

Steatorrhea: The presence of excess fat in the stool.

Stenosis: A stricture, or narrowing; in Crohn's disease, often a narrowing of the bowel.

Stoma: The surgically created opening where the intestine or colon meets the skin in an ileostomy or colostomy, respectively.

Stricture: A narrowed area of intestine usually caused by scar tissue.

Strictureplasty: An operation to open up an intestinal stricture.

Suppository: A small plug of medicine, often cylindrical, that is inserted into the vagina or anus, and is designed to melt at body temperature.

Systemic: A process that involves the whole body, as opposed to a localized process; for example, fatigue is a systemic symptom, whereas lower back pain is a local symptom.

Thalassemia: An inherited blood disorder that can cause anemia.

Thrush: Oral (mouth and throat) fungal infection; appears as a whitish plaque on the tongue and on the inside lining of the mouth.

TNF: Tumor necrosis factor; this protein plays a central role in the initiation of inflammation in IBD. First described in the setting of tumors, we now know that TNF is commonly found in many inflammatory conditions.

TPN (total parenteral nutrition): Nutrition supplied intravenously.

Tumor: An abnormal growth of tissue; can be benign or malignant.

Ulcerative colitis: A disease characterized by chronic inflammation of the colon.

Ultrasound: A radiologic study that uses sound waves to examine abdominal and pelvic organs; commonly used to look for gallstones and obstruction of the bile duct.

Upper endoscopy: A procedure in which a small, thin, flexible, lighted tube with a camera on the end is passed through the mouth into the esophagus, stomach, and duodenum; an excellent test to detect inflammation and strictures in the upper gastrointestinal tract that allows a biopsy to be taken.

Upper GI series/upper GI series with small bowel follow-through: A radiologic examination of the esophagus, stomach, duodenum, and small bowel. The patient drinks a thick, white liquid shake of barium, and then the barium is tracked by taking X-rays as it travels through the gastrointestinal tract. This is an excellent test to detect strictures, fistulas, and inflammation in the stomach and small bowel.

Uveitis: Inflammation of the uvea, which is the central part of the eye (the iris is part of the uvea).

X-ray: A radiologic study that provides an image of bodily structures.

Index